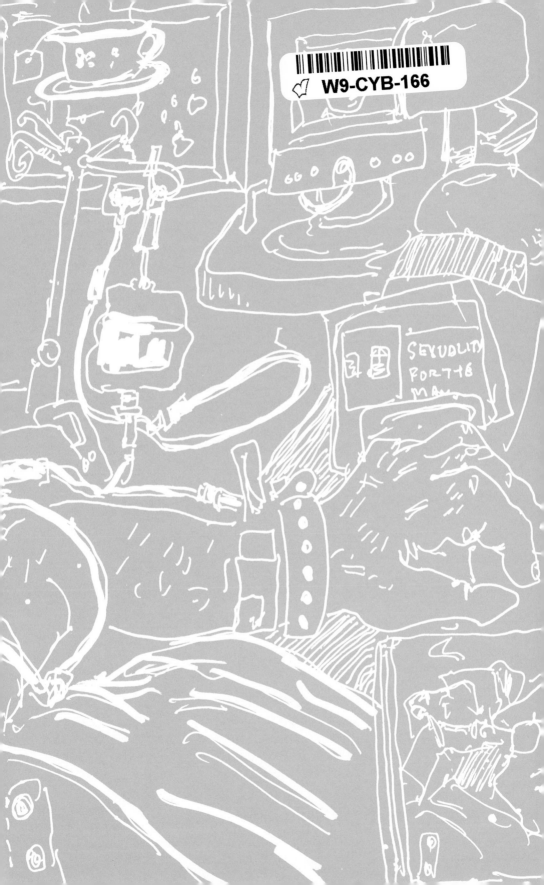

RELATIVELY
INDOLENT
BUT
RELENTLESS

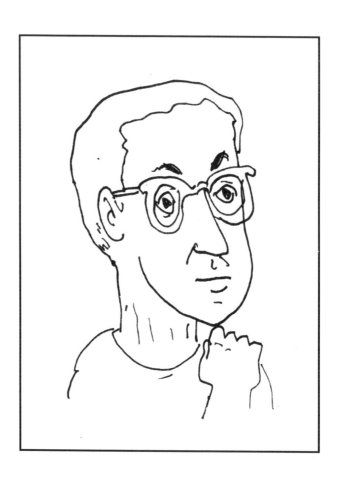

RELATIVELY INDOLENT BUT RELENTLESS

A CANCER TREATMENT JOURNAL

MATT FREEDMAN

SEVEN STORIES PRESS
NEW YORK

SEVEN STORIES PRESS
140 WATTS STREET
NEW YORK, NY 10013
WWW.SEVENSTORIES.COM

COLLEGE PROFESSORS MAY ORDER EXAMINATION COPIES
OF SEVEN STORIES PRESS TITLES FOR FREE. TO ORDER,
VISIT HTTP://WWW.SEVENSTORIES.COM/TEXTBOOK OR SEND
A FAX ON SCHOOL LETTERHEAD TO (212) 226-1411

LIBRARY OF CONGRESS
CATALOGING-IN-PUBLICATION DATA

FREEDMAN, MATT.

RELATIVELY INDOLENT BUT RELENTLESS: A CANCER
TREATMENT JOURNAL / MATT FREEDMAN.— A SEVEN
STORIES PRESS FIRST EDITION. PAGES CM
ISBN 978-1-60980-516-6 (HARDBACK)
1. FREEDMAN, MATT-HEALTH. 2. ADENOID CYSTIC CARCINOMA
— PATIENTS-BIOGRAPHY. 3. HEAD-CANCER-TREATMENT.
4. NECK-CANCER-TREATMENT. 1. TITLE.
RC 280. H4. F74 2014
616.99'4910092-DC23
[B]
                              2013036827

PRINTED IN CHINA
9 8 7 6 5 4 3 2 1

PREFACE

THIS BOOK REPRODUCES A JOURNAL I KEPT IN THE FALL OF 2012 WHILE I WAS UNDERGOING CARE AT MASSACHUSETTS GENERAL HOSPITAL FOR ADENOID CYSTIC CARCINOMA, A RARE CANCER THAT HAD SPREAD FROM MY TONGUE TO MY NECK AND LUNGS BY THE TIME IT WAS DIAG- NOSED. FRIENDS GAVE ME A SKETCHBOOK BEFORE I LEFT FOR BOSTON, AND I DECIDED I WOULD GRADUALLY FILL THE THING UP WITH WHATEVER CAME INTO MY HEAD DURING THE COURSE OF MY TREATMENT.

I WAS FACING AROUND SEVEN WEEKS OF RADIATION AND CHEMOTHERAPY. IF I COMPLETED JUST FOUR PAGES A DAY, I WOULD FILL THE ENTIRE 240-PAGE BOOK BY THE TIME I WAS DONE. THAT LOOKED LIKE A GOOD TRADE - A NOTE- BOOK FILLED WITH WORDS AND PICTURES IN EXCHANGE FOR SIMPLY LIVING THROUGH AN UNAVOIDABLE ORDEAL. EVEN IF I HAD NOTHING WORTHWHILE TO SAY ON MY OWN, I FIGURED I WOULD AT LEAST HAVE A RELATIVELY UNVARNISHED AND RELIABLE RECORD OF WHAT WAS SURE TO BE AN INTERESTING EXPERIENCE.

COMPLETING THE TREATMENT AND COM-
PLETING THE BOOK TOOK MUCH THE SAME
KIND OF UNDERWHELMING COMMITMENT:
DAY-TO-DAY INCREMENTAL PROGRESS THAT
LED TO FINAL RESULTS THAT WERE IM-
POSSIBLE TO IMAGINE AT THE BEGINNING

I BEGAN EVERY PAGE WITH NO IDEA OF
HOW I WOULD FILL IT UP. I JUST LET THE
WORDS AND IMAGES CIRCLE AROUND
EACH OTHER. I DISCOVERED THAT THE
FORM THE JOURNAL TOOK, HANDWRITTEN
NOTES AND FAST DRAWINGS CONFINED TO
A HIGHLY RESTRICTED PHYSICAL SPACE,
HAD A TREMENDOUSLY LIMITING EFFECT
ON WHAT I WROTE AND DREW. I COULD
NOT AFFORD TO GO OFF ON FLIGHTS
OF FANCY BECAUSE I HAD NO CONFIDENCE
THAT I COULD WRITE MY WAY OUT OF A
CORNER WITHOUT SO MANY AMENDMENTS
THAT THE PAGE WOULD BECOME INCOHERENT.
I HAD TO LITERALLY LOOK AHEAD AS I WROTE
AS WELL, WEIGHING AND MEASURING MY WORDS
WITH CARE, FEELING FOR THE BOTTOM OF
THE PAGE AND ANTICIPATING WHERE AND
HOW THE DRAWINGS AND DIAGRAMS WOULD
FIT INTO THE EVOLVING LAYOUT. THIS SEVERE-
LY RESTRICTED STRUCTURE PROBABLY HELPED
ME FINISH THE PROJECT, BUT I DID NOT ANTI-
CIPATE THAT ANY COHERENT NARRATIVE
WOULD EMERGE FROM EACH DAY'S STRESSFUL

SESSION, OR EVEN THAT THE CONTENTS OF THE BOOK WOULD RESONATE WITH ANYONE WHO DIDN'T KNOW ME PERSONALLY.

AS MY TREATMENTS PILED UP AND I BECAME INCREASINGLY INCAPACITATED THE COHERENCE OF MY RECORD BECAME SOMEWHAT COMPROMISED, BUT WE HAVE DONE LITTLE TO ALTER THE ORIGINAL JOURNAL HERE OTHER THAN TO TRY TO MAKE THE PAGES AND TEXT SLIGHTLY MORE LEGIBLE.

THE ONE THING I DO KNOW FOR SURE IS THAT ABSOLUTELY NONE OF THIS WOULD BE POSSIBLE WITHOUT THE LOVING CARE OF MY REMARKABLE FAMILY AND FRIENDS, WHO HUMBLE ME AND TEND TO THE FEARS OF MY SKEPTICAL HEART EVERY DAY.

FOR MORE INFORMATION ON ADENOID CYSTIC CARCINOMA, PLEASE VISIT THE WEB SITES OF TWO WONDERFUL ORGANIZATIONS, THE ADENOID CYSTIC CARCINOMA RESEARCH FOUNDATION AT ACCRF.ORG, OR THE ADENOID CYSTIC CARCINOMA ORGANIZATION INTERNATIONAL AT ACCOI.ORG.

Matt Freedman

RIDGEWOOD, QUEENS
SEPTEMBER, 2013

FOR RADIANT JUDE

NOTES

1. JOSH BRAIN
2. GOLEM
3. CLUMPISM
4. ACME ACME
5. FUNERARY URNS
6. JUDE MEET
7. THUMB
8. BELL
9. WHO I LOOK LIKE
10. TIMELINE OF DEATH
11. MASK
12. HALLOWEEN IN CHI
13. Stas 2
14. WHAT LEETHE
15. VANITY — look
16. speaking like a child
17. schmidt porr accent
18. Grandma forgoly
19. INVERSE PROPORTION OF VANITY
20. JIVE EYENESS FROM JUDE
21. Still hfc pills
22. eating/sleeping realm
23. Harvard pulls me Boston
24. Jacks
    Fuss
    meta-boy
    hole in stud
    MARRIAGE DISSOLUTION AS SCULPT
    some Guys
    mime matt
    CANCER MANHATTAN
    CHURCH LADY
    NECK BETTER — WOLVERINE
    BOYE BDK SIM
    JUDE: WONDERFULNESS
    "How small everything
    IS"
    How much energy
    work slug
    FRUITLAND

YESTERDAY MY COLLEAGUES AND STUDENTS GAVE ME THIS SKETCH BOOK TO FILL UP OVER ~~FOR~~ THE NEXT TWO MONTHS WHILE I UNDERGO RADIATION AND CHEMO THERAPY. I'M GOING TO GET PROTON RADIATION TO FIGHT THE TUMOR IN MY TONGUE.

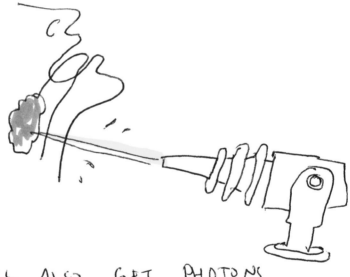

I WILL ALSO GET PHOTONS TO FIGHT THE TUMORS IN MY LYMPH NODES IN MY NECK.

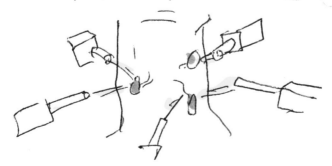

THERE WILL ALSO BE CHEMO-
THERAPY TO SENSITIZE THE
CANCER CELLS. THEY HOPE
THEY WILL GET A "TWO-FER"
OUT OF THE CHEMO AND IT
WILL ALSO ATTACK THE TUMORS
IN MY LUNGS.

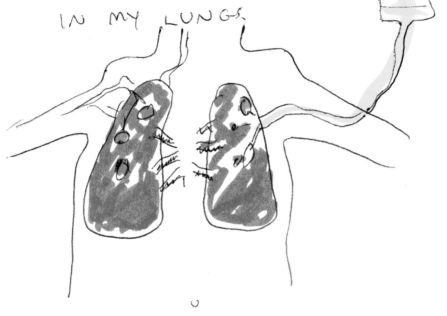

IT'S OCTOBER 3 AND I'VE
KNOWN FOR ABOUT TWO MONTHS
THAT I HAVE ADENOID CYSTIC
CACINOMA, A RARE CANCER
THAT IS "SLOW AND INDOLENT".
IT MOVES SLOWLY BUT IS

HARD TO STOP.
NO ONE KNOWS HOW LONG
THE CANCER HAS BEEN IN
ME IT COULD HAVE BEEN
YEARS.

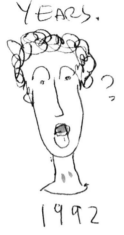

1992

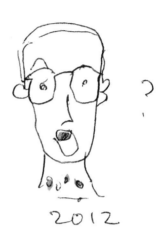

2012

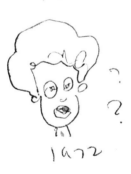

1972

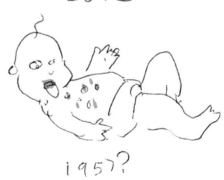

1957?

I'VE HAD A BAD EARACHE
FOR YEARS. FOR MOST OF THAT
TIME I THOUGHT IT WAS CAUSED
BY NIGHT TIME TOOTH GRINDING.

(FELT LIKE A
HOT POKER IN
MY LEFT EAR)

I HAD MOUTH GUARDS MADE
THAT SORT OF
WORKED, BUT
NOT REALLY,
AND NOT FOR
LONG.

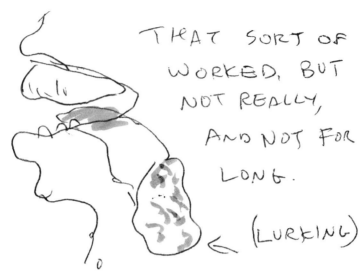

← (LURKING)

AND BESIDES THE DOG ATE
THEM EVERY TIME IT COULD.

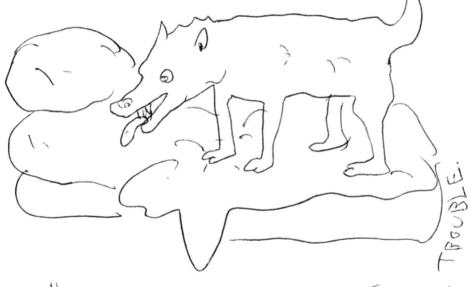

THE TROUBLE.

I'M VERY SLOPPY AND I LET
THINGS GO WHEN I SHOULDN'T.
MAYBE THAT WAS THE ROOT OF ALL

NOW I HAVE A NEW PEN. OCT 4

ABOUT SIX MONTHS AGO
THE PAIN IN MY EAR BEGAN
TO SPREAD TO THE TOP OF MY
HEAD AND DOWN TO MY NECK

EXACTLY TO THE
MIDDLE OF MY HEAD.

IT ALSO BEGAN
TO AFFECT MY
RIGHT EAR
OCCASIONALLY.

THEN I FOUND A BUMP
ON MY NECK.

BUT STILL I ASSUMED IT WAS
ALL BECAUSE OF THE ORIGINAL
EAR ACHE AND THE YEARS
OF CLENCHING MY TEETH.
ANYTHING BUT THAT
WOULD BE TOO COINCIDENTAL
TO BE POSSIBLE AND I DO
NOT BELIEVE IN COINCIDENCES.
I MEAN, I BELIEVE IN
THEM, BUT NOT FOR ME.

I BELIEVE I AM AVERAGE
AND THAT ONLY AVERAGE
THINGS CAN HAPPEN TO ME.
I BEGAN TO FEEL THIS WAY WHEN
I WENT TO MY FIRST BASEBALL
GAME AT THE AGE OF TEN OR SO.

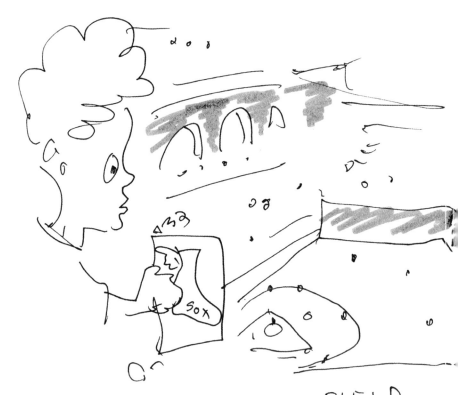

I LOOKED DOWN ON THE FIELD
AND SAW NINE PLAYERS. I LOOKED
AROUND THE PARK AND SAW 50,000
PEOPLE WATCHING THE GAME. I TRIED
TO FIGURE THE CHANCES THAT OUT
OF THE 50,009 PEOPLE IN THE

STADIUM, I WOULD BE ONE OF THE MAJOR LEAGUERS ON THE FIELD. THE ODDS WEREN'T GREAT. I THINK I GAVE UP MY DREAM OF BEING A GREAT BASEBALL PLAYER RIGHT THEN.

I NEVER FOUGHT BACK AGAINST THE ODDS.

WHEN I READ THAT RENOIR SAID HE WAS A CORK IN THE RIVER OF LIFE, I DECIDED RIGHT THEN THAT WAS FOR ME. NO DECISIONS! AND HE WAS AN ARTIST PEOPLE SAID WAS GREAT TO BOOT.

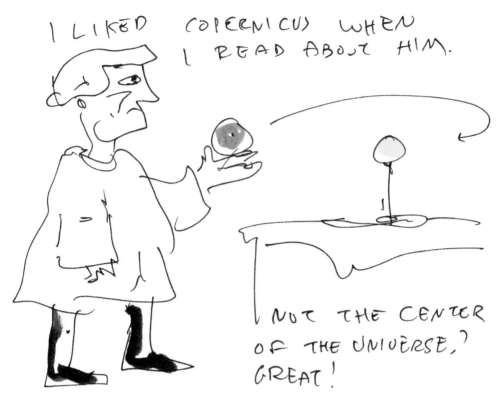

I LIKED COPERNICUS WHEN
I READ ABOUT HIM.

NOT THE CENTER
OF THE UNIVERSE,?
GREAT!

NOT IN THE MIDDLE OF AN
EXCITING PERIOD OF CHANGE
IN THE HISTORY OF THE
UNIVERSE? SOUNDS REASONABLE.

THE POINT IS, I NEVER REALLY
THOUGHT I WOULD BE SINGLED
OUT FOR ANYTHING REMARKABLE.

I WENT TO A SCHOOL WHERE
EVERYBODY WAS SMART.

EVERYBODY WAS IN THE TOP 1%
OF ALL TESTS. SO EVEN BEING
EXCEPTIONAL WAS ORDINARY

(NORMAL) (LAB SCHOOL)

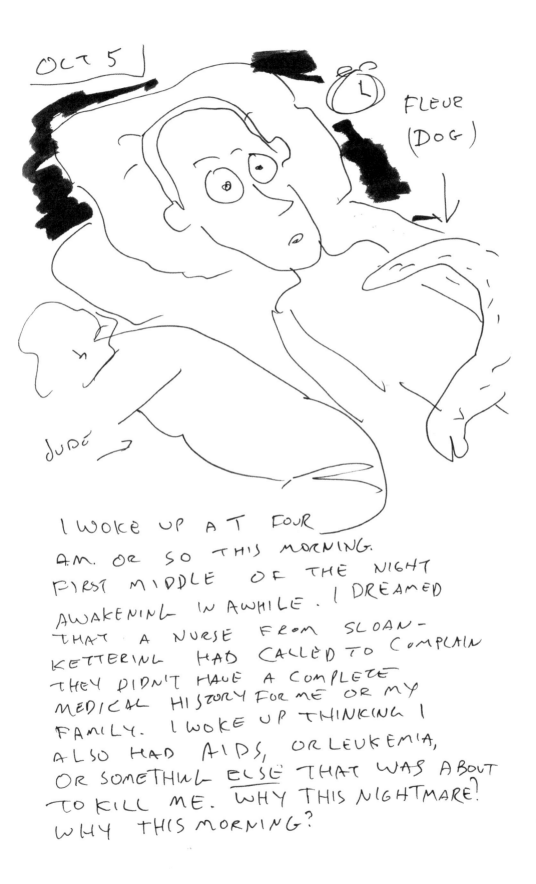

OCT 5

FLEUR
(DOG)

JUDE

I WOKE UP AT FOUR
A.M. OR SO THIS MORNING.
FIRST MIDDLE OF THE NIGHT
AWAKENING IN AWHILE. I DREAMED
THAT A NURSE FROM SLOAN-
KETTERING HAD CALLED TO COMPLAIN
THEY DIDN'T HAVE A COMPLETE
MEDICAL HISTORY FOR ME OR MY
FAMILY. I WOKE UP THINKING I
ALSO HAD AIDS, OR LEUKEMIA,
OR SOMETHING ELSE THAT WAS ABOUT
TO KILL ME. WHY THIS NIGHTMARE?
WHY THIS MORNING?

A FRIEND WROTE AN EMAIL
LAST NIGHT EXPRESSING CONDOLENCES
FOR THE "**HORROR**" I WAS UNDERGOING

I DIDN'T THINK MUCH OF IT
AT THE TIME, BUT I THINK THAT
STARTED A TICKING TIME BOMB
THAT WENT OFF IN THE MIDDLE
OF THE NIGHT.

CORNUCOPIA

IN THE LAST FEW WEEKS I'VE
STARTED CALMING DOWN AND THINKING
I HAD THINGS UNDER CONTROL. GOT

FIGHT WITH
INSURANCE
COMPANY
(WON)

DECIDE
WHERE TO
HAVE RADIATION
(EMPOWERING)

GET PLACE TO
STAY (THANK YOU,
ELLEN)

I HAD STOPPED THINKING ABOUT DYING, JUST TRYING TO KEEP UP WITH THE BUSINESS OF BEING SICK WAS A FULL TIME JOB. NOW THE HORROR WAS BACK, AT LEAST FOR A MIDDLE OF THE NIGHT VISIT. I'VE ALWAYS LIKED HORROR MOVIES. THE OLD FASHIONED KIND AT LEAST.

JUICING MACHINE

GET MASK

THERE WAS A LOT TO DO AND IT DISTRACTED ME FROM BEING SICK IN THE FIRST PLACE.

THERE WAS CREATURE
FEATURES, ON OLD TV.

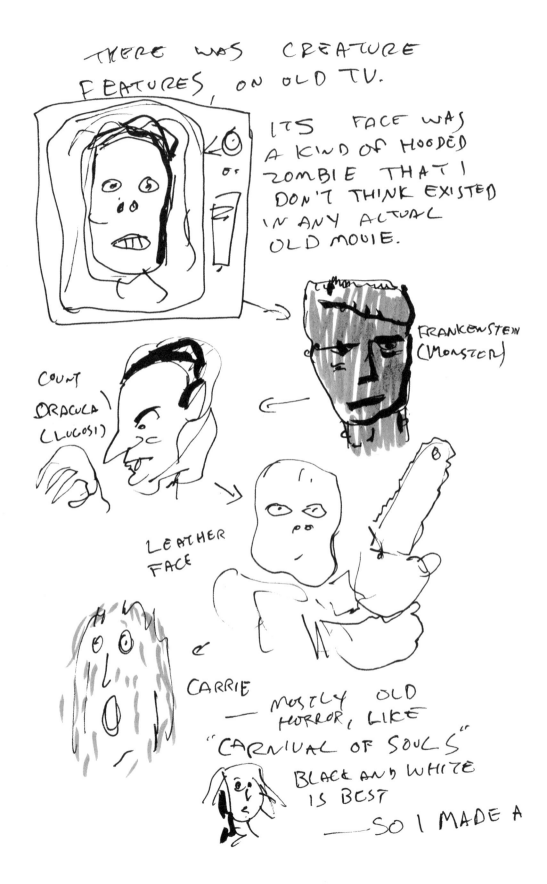

ITS FACE WAS
A KIND OF HOODED
ZOMBIE THAT I
DON'T THINK EXISTED
IN ANY ACTUAL
OLD MOVIE.

FRANKENSTEIN
(MONSTER)

COUNT
DRACULA
(LUGOSI)

LEATHER
FACE

CARRIE

MOSTLY OLD
HORROR, LIKE
"CARNIVAL OF SOULS"
BLACK AND WHITE
IS BEST
—SO I MADE A

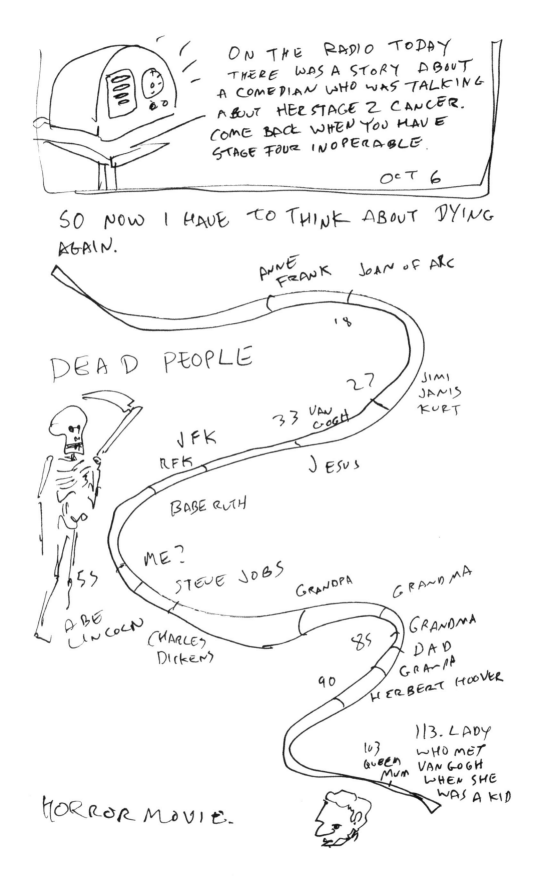

TOMORROW I DRIVE UP TO BOSTON
AND I START CHEMO AND RADIATION
WEDNESDAY.
  I WORRY ABOUT:
  1. BUS SYSTEM
  2. LAUNDRY
  3. PAIN IN NECK AND HEAD
  4. ENTERTAINING GUESTS

THE HORROR MOVIE WAS SUPPOSED
TO BE ABOUT A GIRL FROM THE
POLISH TOWN OF AUSCHWITZ WHO
MOVES TO NYC TO BECOME A FOLK SINGER
AND MOVES INTO A SYNAGOGUE. THIS
IS TRUE.

OUR FRIEND
ELA MOVED
IN TO OUR
HOUSE WHICH
IS AN OLD
SYNAGOGUE.

ONCE
THERE,
SHE MEETS
TWO
OLD LADIES.

RUTH

PERLENE

THEY EXIST TOO.

IN THE MOVIE,
THEY ARE
GHOSTS

SHE IS MOVING IN TO TAKE
INVENTORY OF THE WORK OF TWO
ARTISTS WHO WERE KILLED IN
THEIR STUDIO WHEN THEY FELL OFF THEIR
LADDERS WHILE FIXING A STAINED GLASS WINDOW.

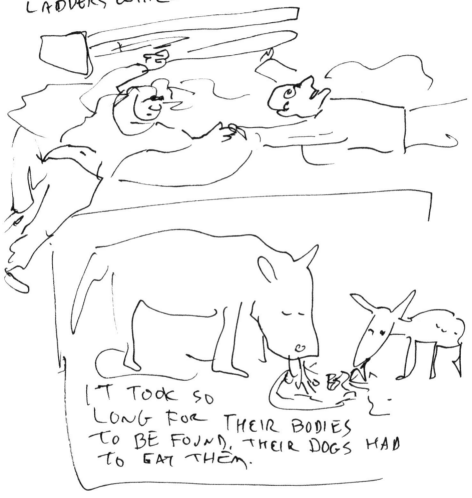

IT TOOK SO
LONG FOR THEIR BODIES
TO BE FOUND, THEIR DOGS HAD
TO EAT THEM.

SHE FEELS SO GUILTY ABOUT
BEING FROM AUSCHWITZ THAT
WE DON'T KNOW IF SHE IS CRAZY
OR NOT. SHE THINKS SHE HAS
MET A GOLEM.

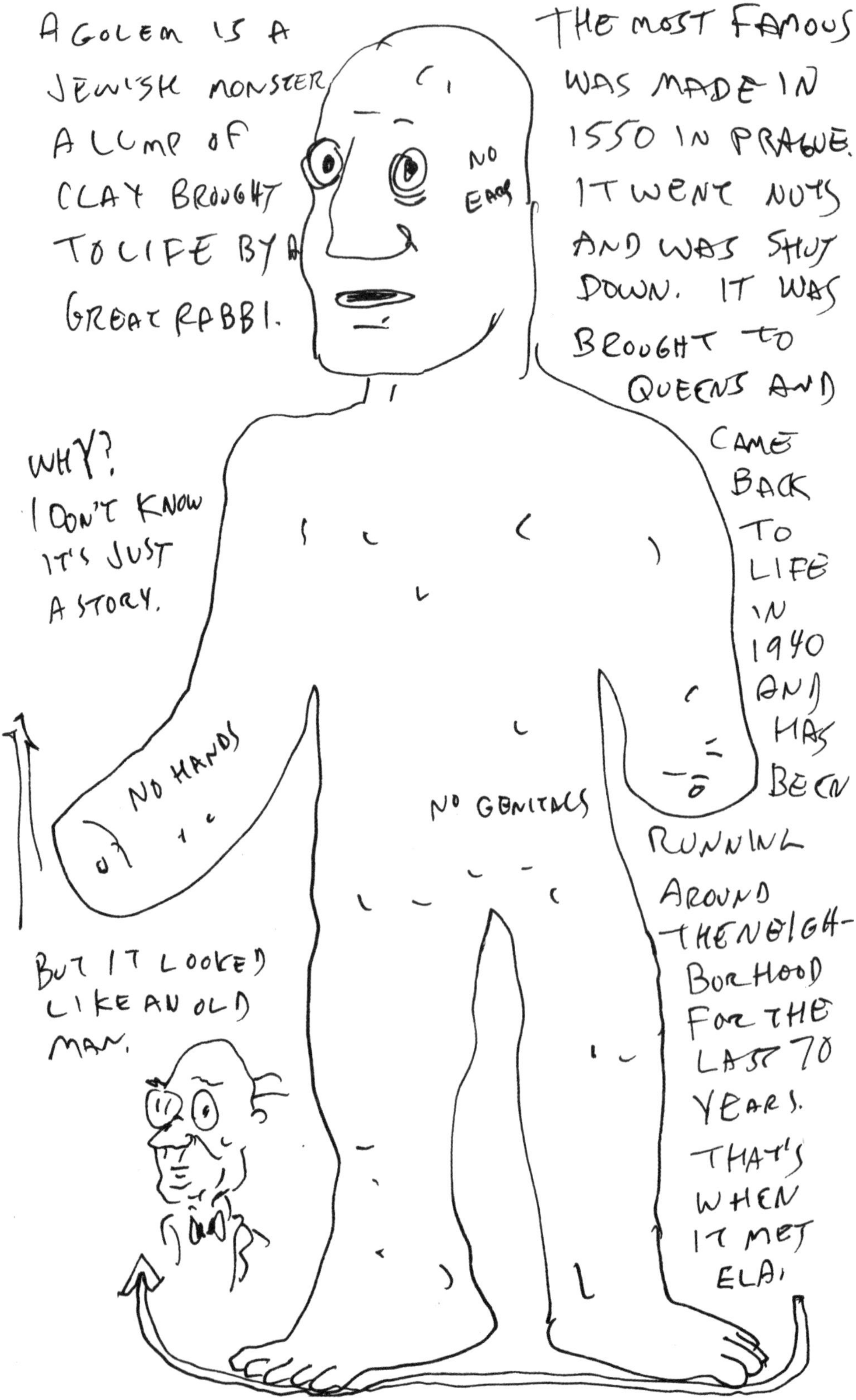
A GOLEM IS A JEWISH MONSTER A LUMP OF CLAY BROUGHT TO LIFE BY A GREAT RABBI.
THE MOST FAMOUS WAS MADE IN 1550 IN PRAGUE. IT WENT NUTS AND WAS SHUT DOWN. IT WAS BROUGHT TO QUEENS AND
NO EARS
WHY? I DON'T KNOW IT'S JUST A STORY.
CAME BACK TO LIFE IN 1940 AND HAS BEEN
NO HANDS
NO GENITALS
RUNNING AROUND THE NEIGH-BORHOOD FOR THE LAST 70 YEARS.
BUT IT LOOKED LIKE AN OLD MAN.
THAT'S WHEN IT MET ELAI

WHAT HAPPENED THOUGH WAS OCT 7
THAT I LEARNED I WASN'T A PROPER
DIRECTOR. I HAD A HARD TIME ORGANIZING
THINGS AND I COULDN'T TELL PEOPLE
WHAT TO DO. SO I PUT THE SCREEN PLAY
ON A SHELF. THIS HAD HAPPENED SO
MANY TIMES I HAD A COLLECTION OF
MANUSCRIPTS BOLTED INTO SCULPTURES

1983-86
"BRUCE
TAKES
HIS TIME"
(NOVEL)

1987-88
"AWFUL"
NOVEL

100
SHORT STORIES
IN 100
DAYS:
JACK CORONA
VS. BRUNO
CARNICIOUS

1983

[4a]
"THE ANTIQUE
A BOMB *"
SCREEN
PLAY

* I DON'T REMEMBER
THE REAL
TITLE

"WILLIAMSBURG
STORY *"
NOVEL

* I DON'T
REMEMBER
THE REAL TITLE

1999

"THE BENEFITS
OF DOUBT"
NOVEL

2000?

"24 HOURS *"

NOVEL

* I DON'T
REMEMBER
THE REAL
TITLE

"THE
GOLEM
OF RIDGEWOOD"
2010-2011

(AND THERE WERE OTHERS)   ALL MANUSCRIPTS
WERE BOLTED INSIDE
CAST FIGURES

SO THIS EVENING IS THE FIRST
IN BOSTON. NOW THINGS WILL FINALLY
START TO HAPPEN. I'VE LEFT HOME
TO START TREATMENT.

LAST NIGHT JUST BEFORE WE WENT
OUT TO HAVE A LAST DINNER WITH
FRIENDS THE DOG STARTED FRANTICALLY
SCRATCHING AT THE DOOR.

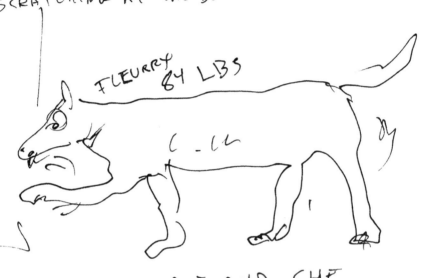

FLEURRY 84 LBS

SO I LET HER OUT AND SHE
RAN UP THE STEPS.

SIDE YARD

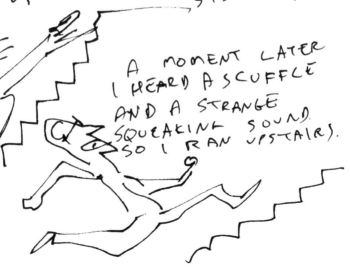

A MOMENT LATER
I HEARD A SCUFFLE
AND A STRANGE
SQUEAKING SOUND.
SO I RAN UPSTAIRS.

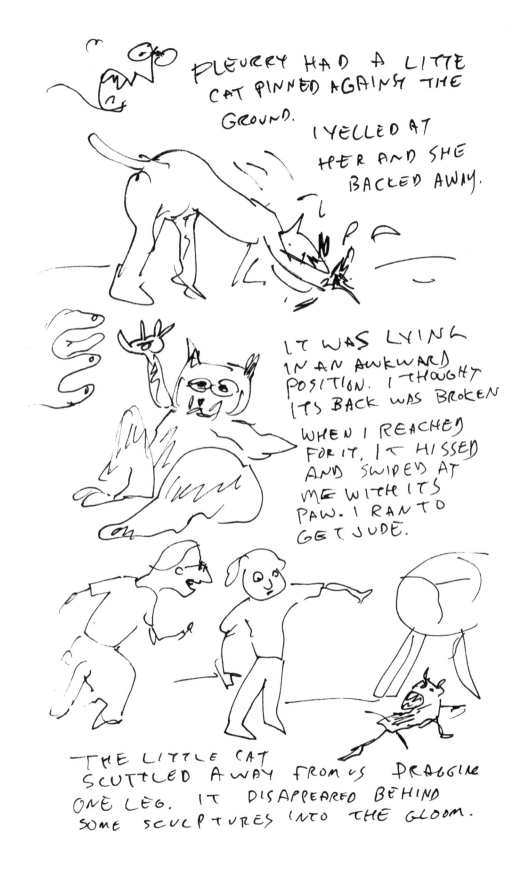

PLEURRY HAD A LITTLE
CAT PINNED AGAINST THE
GROUND. I YELLED AT
HER AND SHE
BACKED AWAY.

IT WAS LYING
IN AN AWKWARD
POSITION. I THOUGHT
ITS BACK WAS BROKEN

WHEN I REACHED
FOR IT, IT HISSED
AND SWIPED AT
ME WITH ITS
PAW. I RAN TO
GET JUDE.

THE LITTLE CAT
SCUTTLED AWAY FROM US DRAGGING
ONE LEG. IT DISAPPEARED BEHIND
SOME SCULPTURES INTO THE GLOOM.

WE RAN AROUND TO THE FRONT OF THE
BUILDING WITH A CAT CARRIER AND
A TOWEL. WE THOUGHT WE COULD
CATCH IT AND TAKE IT TO AN
ANIMAL HOSPITAL AND SAVE IT.

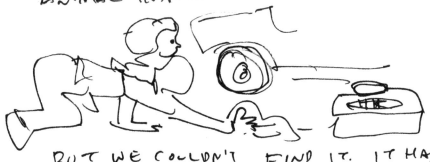

BUT WE COULDN'T FIND IT. IT HAD
DISAPPEARED. WE CAN ONLY HOPE
IT HAD A QUICK AND RELATIVELY
PAINLESS DEATH.

THIS WAS A TERRIBLE WAY
TO BEGIN THE WEEK.
I SHOULD HAVE STOPPED THE
DOG. I SHOULD HAVE SAVED
THE CAT. I SHOULD HAVE
PUT THE CAT OUT OF ITS
MISERY. INSTEAD, I STOOD
AROUND AND DID NOTHING UNTIL
IT WAS TOO LATE.
I ALWAYS WAIT TOO LONG.

THE DOG PLAYS
WITH OUR TWO CATS
BUT IT KILLS WILD
CATS, BIRDS + SQUIRRELS.

BUS | COLU

THE BANKS AND THE HOSPITAL ~~AND~~ FINANCIAL OFFICES WERE CLOSED TODAY FOR COLUMBUS' BIRTHDAY. I DID NOT GET TO FIGURE OUT MONEY SITUATION.

WENT OVER TO SEE HOUSE WHERE I WILL STAY DURING TREATMENT. MY FRIEND ELLEN HAD BEEN STAYING THERE BEFORE SHE MOVED AWAY TO HAVE SPACE FOR HER DOGS + CATS + HORSES.

SHE HAD HER TWO DOGS WITH HER.

ROLLIE

PIPPA

WHILE WE WERE OUTSIDE THIS AFTERNOON, PIPPA KILLED A YOUNG SQUIRREL.

TONIGHT I AM STAYING IN
APARTMENT. IT IS PRETTY FULL

THE FRONT ROOM OF THE
OF STUFF
ITS ALSO LIGHT
FILLED
AND
COZY.

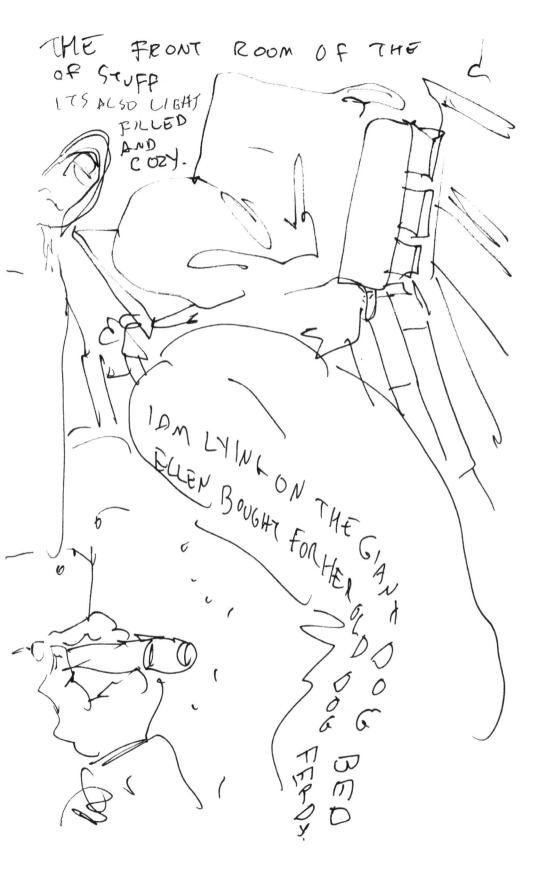

I AM LYING ON THE GIANT
ELLEN BOUGHT FOR HER OLD DOG DOG BED FERDY.

ELLEN TOLD ME ABOUT A
CONVERSATION SHE HAD WITH
A HORSE OF HERS AFTER IT
DIED.

IT SAID IT HAD
LIKED THE BEST
HOME IT HAD LIVED
AT FOR RETIRED
SHOW HORSES

BECAUSE ALL
THE HORSES THERE
HAD BEEN TREATED
WITH RESPECT AND
THERE HAD BEEN NO
STARS.

THE HORSE HAD
HAD A PRETTY HIGH
OPINION OF ITSELF,
SO IT SAID A LOT THAT
IT HAD FELT THE
RETIREMENT HOME'S
"NO STARS" POLICY
HAD SOMETHING GOING FOR IT.

YOU CAN ONLY COMMUNICATE WITH
DEAD ANIMALS FOR A SHORT TIME
AFTER THEIR DEATHS. AFTER THAT
THEY GET HARDER AND HARDER TO
FIND AND YOU LOSE CONTACT.

SO TOMORROW EVERYTHING [OCT 9
STARTS. I'VE GOTTEN FOND OF
THE ACHE IN MY HEAD ANY
EAR OVER THE LAST FEW MONTHS.
BEFORE THE DIAGNOSIS, WHEN THEY
WERE ANNOYING PAINS, THE SENSATIONS
SEEMED TRIVIAL AND SILLY. NOW THAT
I KNOW HOW DIRE THE REASONS
BEHIND THEM ARE, THEY ARE
WORTHY COMPANIONS THAT GIVE MEANING
TO LIFE.

THE LEFT SIDE OF THE
HEAD OCCASIONALLY
ALL ACHES IN
ONE BIG SUPER
CONTINENT OF
SORENESS FROM
THE TOP OF THE
HEAD TO THE CLAVICLE.
THE RIGHT
EAR PIPES
UP EVERY NOW
AND THEN.

THE TELL-
TALE EAR
PAIN COMES
AND GOES
THE DRUGS
HELP

THE
LEFT EYE
HAS A FEELING
OF PRESSURE
ALWAYS. NOT
UN PLEASANT

The swollen node
is painless UNLESS
PRESSED, THEN IT
ACHES FOR
A FEW
HOURS

BUT LIKE IT JUST MIGHT POP OUT
SOME DAY!

PRESSURE ON RIB CAGE AROUND LUNGS
EVER SINCE DIAGNOSIS +
BIOPSY.

WHAT I WONDER IS IF THE
THERAPY WILL ACTUALLY MAKE THE
PAIN GO AWAY - OR JUST CURE THE CANCER.
OR JUST CURE THE CANCER AND
NOT MAKE THE PAIN GO AWAY.
OR NEITHER.
FOR YEARS I THINK I HESITATED
ABOUT GOING FOR TREATMENT FOR
THE PAIN BECAUSE I ACTUALLY TOOK
COMFORT FROM THE POSSIBILITY THAT
A SOLUTION MIGHT BE POSSIBLE.
ALMOST LIKE BUYING A LOTTERY
TICKET GIVES YOU THE SENSATION
OF BEING RICH EVEN IF IT CAN'T
MAKE YOU RICH.

LOTTERY
0 1937651 6

I EVENTUALLY TRIED ACUPUNCTURE
BUT THAT DIDN'T WORK. I DIDN'T
FOLLOW ALL THE DOCTOR'S EATING
ADVICE THOUGH.

BEER
NO

WINE
YES

EMPTY

I DID GO TO AN
ENT DOCTOR ONCE
YEARS AGO — NOBODY
KNOWS WHO OR WHEN —
BECAUSE OF THE PAIN,
BUT HE FOUND NOTHING.

IS IT BETTER TO KNOW?

MY BROTHER, THE DOCTOR
HAD HIS BRAIN SCANNED ON
AN MRI MACHINE A FEW YEARS
AGO TO HELP WITH RESEARCH
HE WAS DOING ON THE MIND.
WHAT THEY FOUND INSTEAD
WAS INCREDIBLE.

HIS BRAIN
WAS FILLED
WITH GIANT
HOLES

LIQUID

HE SHOULD
HAVE BEEN
SEVERELY
RETARDED.

INSTEAD
HE IS
BRILLIANT.

THE BRAIN HAD REWIRED ITSELF
AROUND THE HOLES AND WAS BETTER
THAN EVER. NOBODY EVEN SUSPECTED.

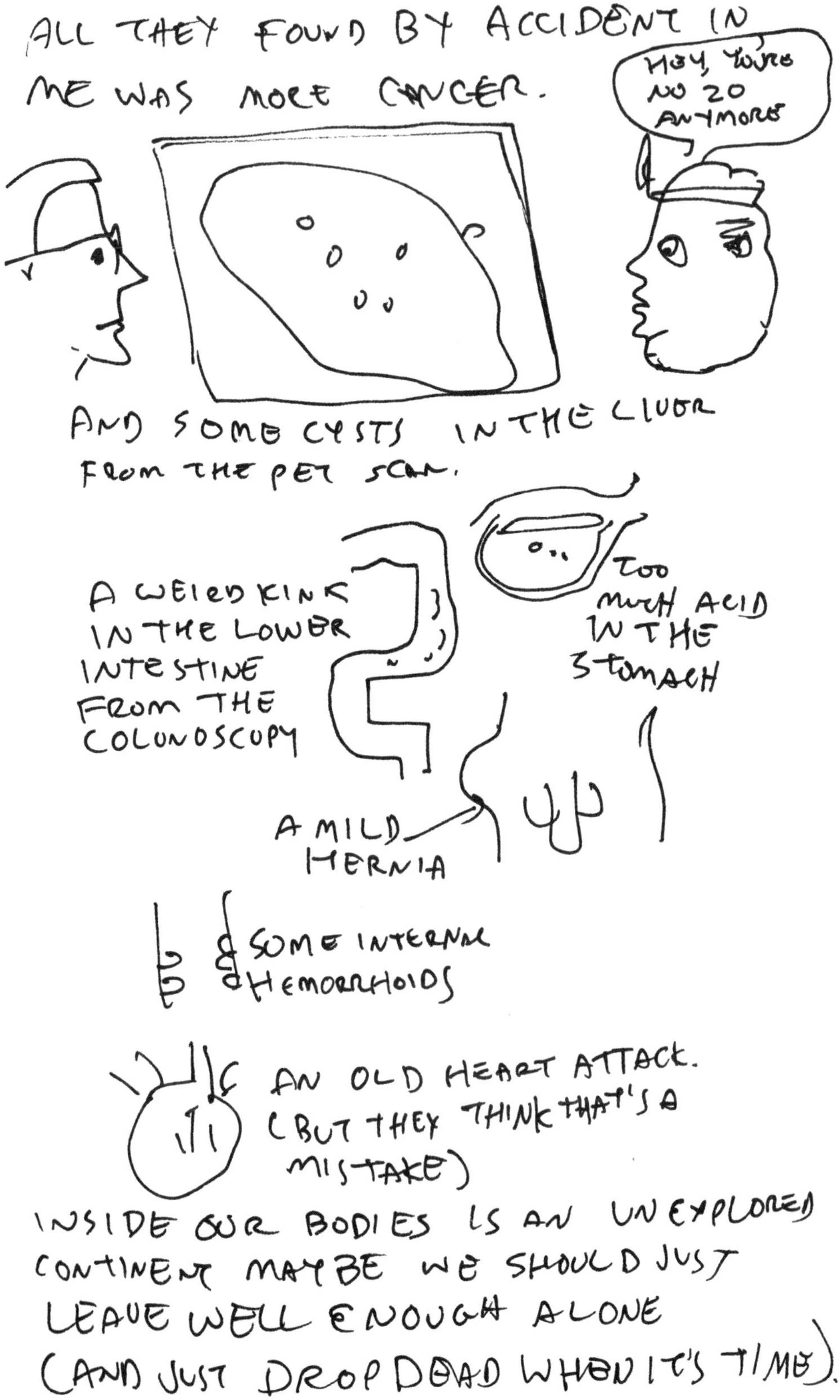
ALL THEY FOUND BY ACCIDENT IN ME WAS MORE CANCER.
HEY, YOU'RE NO 20 ANYMORE
AND SOME CYSTS IN THE LIVER FROM THE PET SCAN.
A WEIRD KINK IN THE LOWER INTESTINE FROM THE COLONOSCOPY
TOO MUCH ACID IN THE STOMACH
A MILD HERNIA
& SOME INTERNAL HEMORRHOIDS
AN OLD HEART ATTACK. (BUT THEY THINK THAT'S A MISTAKE)
INSIDE OUR BODIES IS AN UNEXPLORED CONTINENT MAYBE WE SHOULD JUST LEAVE WELL ENOUGH ALONE (AND JUST DROP DEAD WHEN IT'S TIME).

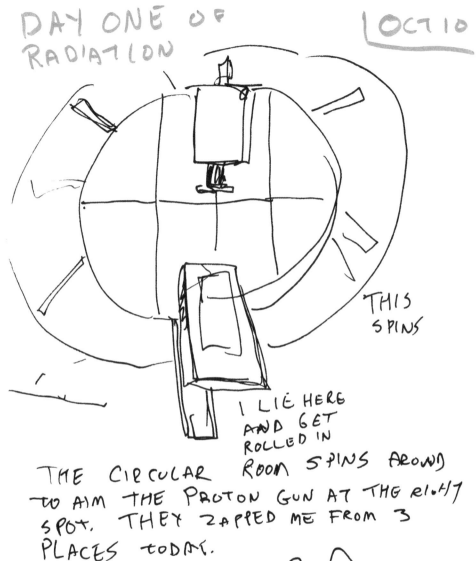

THIS SPINS

I LIE HERE AND GET ROLLED IN

THE CIRCULAR ROOM SPINS AROUND TO AIM THE PROTON GUN AT THE RIGHT SPOT. THEY ZAPPED ME FROM 3 PLACES TODAY.

LEFT SIDE

BELOW

RIGHT SIDE

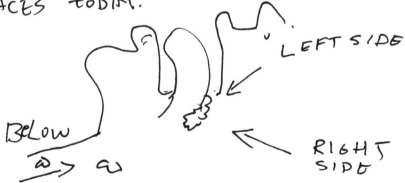

SORT OF THE REVERSE OF THE CANNONS ON THE USS MONITOR. THE TURRET SPUN AND THE 2 CANNONS SHOT 360°

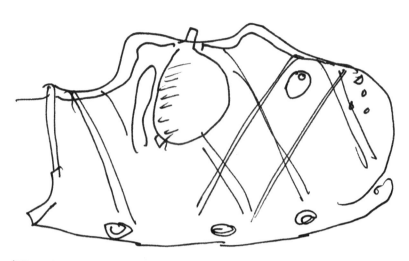

FIRST THEY BOLTED MY SPECIALLY
MADE-FOR-MY-HEAD FACE MASK ON.
ACTUALLY FIRST THEY PUT THE SPECIALLY
MADE FOR MY MOUTH MOUTHPIECE IN
MY MOUTH. IT ALMOST CHOKES ME
AFTER THIRTY MINUTES IN THERE
I FEEL LIKE I'M GOING TO STRANGLE.
I CAN FEEL THE BURN IN MY TONGUE.
I CAN SMELL IT. I'M COOKING.

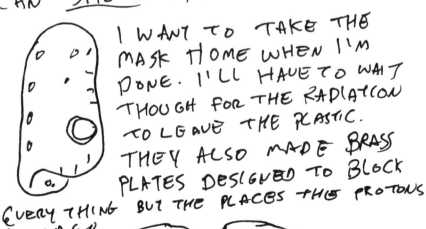

I WANT TO TAKE THE
MASK HOME WHEN I'M
DONE. I'LL HAVE TO WAIT
THOUGH FOR THE RADIATION
TO LEAVE THE PLASTIC.
THEY ALSO MADE BRASS
PLATES DESIGNED TO BLOCK
EVERY THING BUT THE PLACES THE PROTONS
SHOULD GO.

WHEN I AM DONE I HAVE THE WAFFLE PATTERN PRESSED ONTO MY FACE.

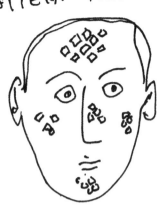

THE WAFFLE MARKS SHOULD FADE.

THE IRRADIATED AREA ON THE NECK AND UNDER THE CHIN MAY NOT FADE. IT MAY BE DARK. IT MAY NOT GROW HAIR. I HAVE TO REMEMBER TO PUT MOISTERIZING OINTMENT ON AND DO MY STRETCHING EXERCISES

EVERY DAY.

OPEN MOUTH WIDE FOR 10 SECONDS, FIVE TIMES

← JAW LEFT 5 TIMES, 2 COUNT

JAW RIGHT → 5 TIMES 2 COUNT

STICK OUT TONGUE 5 TIMES

PULL IN TONGUE 5 TIMES

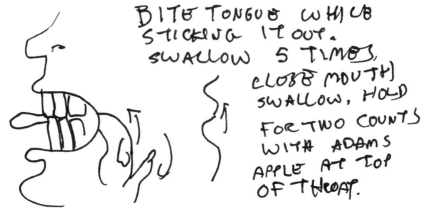

BITE TONGUE WHILE
STICKING IT OUT.
SWALLOW 5 TIMES,
CLOSE MOUTH,
SWALLOW, HOLD
FOR TWO COUNTS
WITH ADAMS
APPLE AT TOP
OF THROAT.

THE IDEA IS TO KEEP THE
TONGUE, NECK AND EPIGLOTIS
FLEXIBLE SO FOOD DOESN'T
FALL DOWN WRONG TUBE INTO
LUNGS.

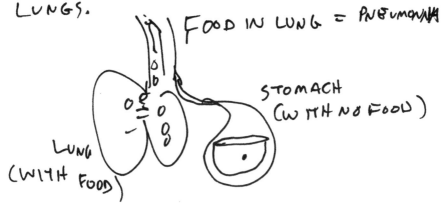

FOOD IN LUNG = PNEUMONIA

STOMACH
(WITH NO FOOD)

LUNG
(WITH FOOD)

THE CURRENT MYSTERY IS SUGAR. WILL
SUGAR KILL ME? WILL NO SUGAR
SAVE ME?

I HATE THAT
THE'RE MIGHT
BE THINGS
ENTIRELY
UNDER MY CONTROL
THAT MAY CONTROL MY
SURVIVAL.

OR

I WANT FATE TO DECIDE EVERY THING.

DRY MOUTH LAST NIGHT. EXCITING.

FIRST SYMPTOMS. | 2 AM | HEADACHE

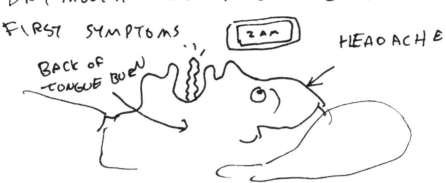

BACK OF
TONGUE BURN

AQUSITON OF THERAPY TOOLS:

FANCY ELECTRIC RAZOR

LESS IRRITATION
NO TEARING OF
SKIN

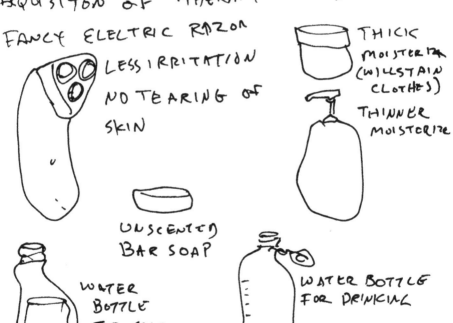

THICK
MOISTERIZ
(WILL STAIN
CLOTHES)

THINNER
MOISTERIZ

UNSCENTED
BAR SOAP

WATER
BOTTLE
FOR SALT +
BAKING SODA
RINSE

WATER BOTTLE
FOR DRINKING

ENERGY BARS   CANDY
                  BAR

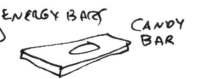

FOLDING TOOTH BRUSH
(THANK YOU MARTINE)

YESTERDAY AFTER THERAPY JUDY
AND I VISITED A BEAUTIFUL BUILDING
MADE AVAILABLE TO CANCER PATIENTS
DURING THERAPY.

BOUNTEOUS GARDENS + CHAIRS
FLOWERS IN AND OUTSIDE

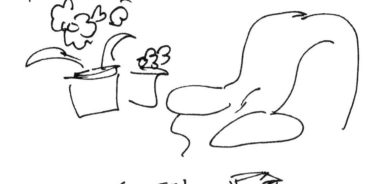

PRIVATE SUITES

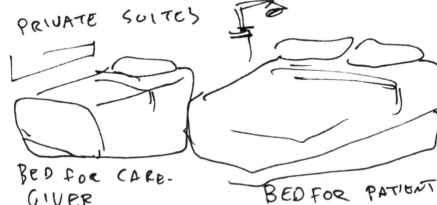

BED FOR CARE-
GIVER

BED FOR PATIENT

HUGE COMMONAL KITCHEN
COUNTER FULL OF TREATS

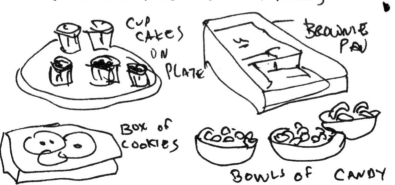

CUP
CAKES
ON
PLATE

BROWNIE
PAN

BOX OF
COOKIES

BOWLS OF CANDY

EVERYWHERE, CANCER PATIENTS

KERCHIEF ON HEAD

REDDISH FLUSH

SWOLLEN FACE

ANGRY BURN MARK

WATTLES

CANE

ALSO, THEY (DRS, RNS, ETC.) START TALKING TO YOU LIKE YOU'RE A CHILD

I'M STILL TOO NEW TO THIS. I'M NOT SEEING MYSELF HERE. I'M STILL A VOYEUR, A POSER, AN INFILTRATOR INTO ANOTHER REALITY. MY HEAD DOES HURT AND MY TONGUE AND MY CHEST. BUT THAT CAN ALL STILL BE IGNORED.

SOMETHING OUT THERE WILL MAKE ME WISE UP. I'M NOT LOOKING FORWARD TO FINDING OUT WHAT THAT WILL BE. NOT LOOKING FORWARD TO SUCH A REVELATION: ODDS ARE 85% IT WILL BE BAD 15% GOOD.

TONIGHT, THE SECOND NIGHT OF RADIATION, THE NECK IS STIFF THE THROAT IS SORE.

THIS AFTERNOON I MET DR WIRTH, THE MEDICAL ONCOLOGIST. SHE TOLD ME I WOULD PROBABLY END UP ON A FEEDING TUBE.

THIS IS NOT WHAT I EXPECTED TO HEAR. THIS IS DISTURBING. IS THIS THE FIRST SIGN OF REAL CANCER?

WHAT HAPPENS IF THE MOUTH DOESN'T WORK? THINK APPARENTLY. THEY DON'T IT'S A BIG DEAL WHAT IF THE

JAW ROTS WITH DISUSE.

TEETH FALL OUT

BONE DIES

JAW AMPUTATED

SKIN PUCKERS. AND THE CANCER KEEPS GROWING. STILL EATING AS MUCH AS ~~____~~. SO THATS GOOD

20^n 6'2" 6'1" 2012

^HUMANLY POSSIBLE. AND I'VE SHRUNK ONE INCH.

LAST NIGHT THINGS GOT BAD
THIS MORNING THEY SEEM BETTER

BIG NEW SYMPTOM LAST NIGHT
WAS VICE-LIKE PRESSURE ON BACK
OF NECK

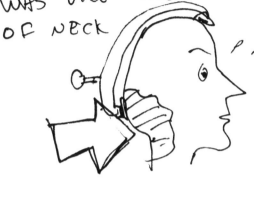

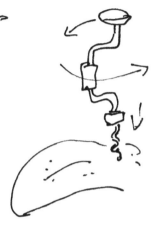

DRILL LIKE
PAIN AT BACK
OF TONGUE

IN THE MIDDLE OF NIGHT THINGS
SEEMED UNENDURABLE AND IT
WAS ONLY THE SECOND NIGHT.
I THOUGHT I WAS TOUGHER.

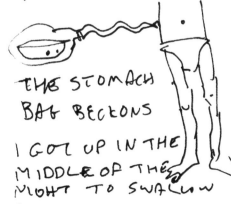

THE STOMACH
BAG BECKONS

I GOT UP IN THE
MIDDLE OF THE
NIGHT TO SWALLOW
PAIN PILLS.

BUT NOW IN
THE MORNING I
FEEL BETTER
TOM IS HERE
HE DID A MORNING
DANCE LIKE HIS
SON NOAH.

PILLS:
DEXAMETHASONE 125 8mg
ACETAMINOPHEN 1000-4000 mg
FISHOIL 1000mg FINE
MAITAKE TBSP ANTI-OXIDENTS MEGA
MULTIVITAMIN - DISCONTINUED
GLUCOSAMINE FINE
HYDROCHORIZIDE 12.5 mL

NO MEGADOSE

FUNGWAH

ON BUS BACK FROM
BOSTON FOR WEEKEND
IN NYC PLANE $ 468
        FAST TRAIN $ 250
        SLOW TRAINS $71-$140
        REGULAR BUS $ 32
        THIS BUS $ IS
(SMELLS LIKE GASOLINE.)
I GUESS THIS PROOF POSITIVE
I'M CHEAP. I WAS BORN
CHEAP AND I'M GOING TO
DIE CHEAP.) (THOUGH I
DID BUY THE MOST EXPENSIVE
ELECTRIC RAZOR IN THE STORE

MY LIST OF DAILY
DRUGS SUBMITTED FOR
INSPECTION. MUSHROOMS
AND MEGAVITAMINS
ARE OUTLAWED.

THE DEXAMETHA-
SONE SHOULD
SPEED ME UP.
CAN'T WAIT
FOR THAT

89.99   79.99   59.99   42.99   25.99
                              (FOR SHAVING
                              BELOW HEAD
                              AND NECK

ALSO I
NON-GENERIC
MOISTERIZERS
BOOGH

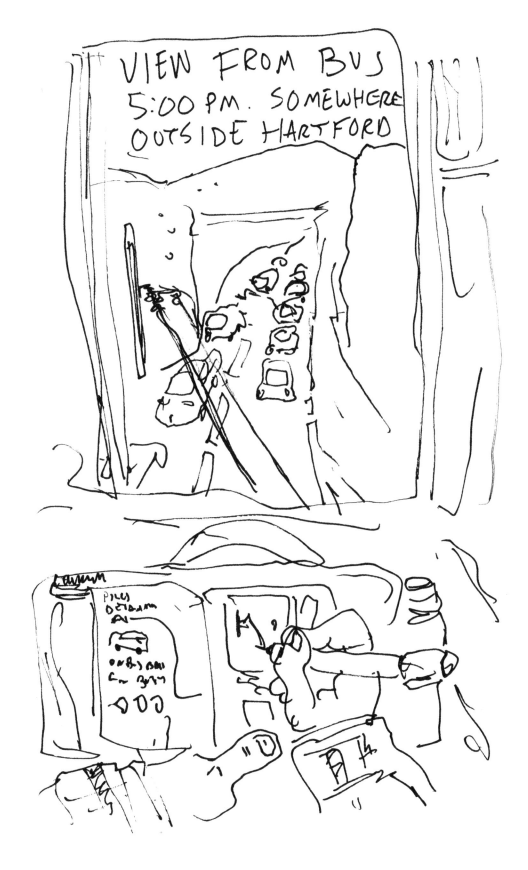

I THINK I'M LOOKING PRETTY
SPIFFY THESE DAYS. AT LEAST I'M
TRYING TO WEAR BETTER CLOTHES
ON THE THEORY THAT AS THE REST
OF ME GOES DOWN HILL, THE SHELL
CAN BE MAINTAINED OR ENHANCED.
BUT MY BROTHER SAYS I BETTER
START SPRUCING UP MORE IF I WANT
THE DOCTORS TO TAKE ME SERIOUSLY.

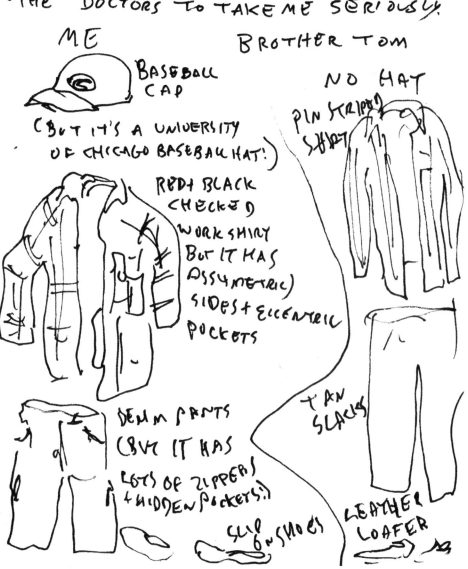

ME

BASEBALL
CAP

(BUT IT'S A UNIVERSITY
OF CHICAGO BASEBALL HAT!)

RED + BLACK
CHECKED
WORK SHIRT
BUT IT HAS
ASSYMETRIC)
SIDES + ECCENTRIC
POCKETS

DENIM PANTS
(BUT IT HAS
LOTS OF ZIPPERS
+ HIDDEN POCKETS!)

SLIP
ON SHOES

BROTHER TOM

NO HAT

PIN STRIPED
SHIRT

TAN
SLACKS

LEATHER
LOAFER

BACK IN NYC LAST NIGHT
JUDE AND I STOPPED AT A SHOW
IN WILLIAMSBURG

OCT 13

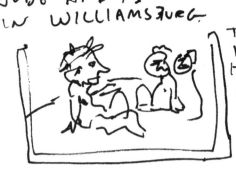

THE ARTIST, KIM JONES
HAD TAKEN DRAWINGS
HE MADE IN 1972
AND DRAWN NEW
IMAGES ON THEM.
ON THE WAY OUT
OF THE GALLERY
MY FRIEND BOB PRESSED A $50
BILL INTO MY HAND AND TOLD
ME TO GO HAVE DINNER.
SO WE DID.

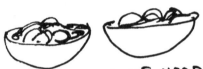

TWO BOWLS OF NOODLES   13.50 EACH

   3.00 + 3.00

DUMPLINGS   KIM CHI   3.00

MOOCHI ICE CREAM   36.00

            TAX   6.25

                                  42.25

50.00   TIP   7.75

                                  50.00

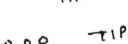
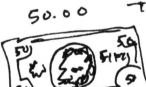
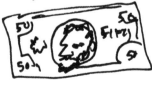

EASY COME EASY GO. THANKS BOB

CATS + DOG HAPPY TO HAVE CLAN BACK

I'M GOING UP TO STUDIO PAPER MACHÉ CORNUCOPIA MONSTER FOR DEC. SHOW IT WON'T DRY. NOW IT WON'T BE READY.

I'M NOTICING SOMETHING: THERE'S NOT AS MUCH TIME AS I THOUGHT THERE WOULD BE FOR REFLECTION AND INSIGHT. I'M STILL AS SHALLOW AS BEFORE. MY FRIEND JON, WHO WENT THROUGH WORSE THAN THIS, WARNED ME ABOUT THAT. ALL ART PROJECTS AND AMBITIOUS HUMAN EXPERIENCES FAIL TO DELIVER ON EXPECTATIONS.

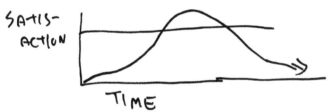

SATIS-ACTION

TIME

AT SOME POINT IN EVERY ARTISTIC PRACTICE THE ARTIST REALIZES THAT THE POWERS THAT BE, THE POWERS THAT DISPENSE TALENT AND ACHIEVEMENT, HAVE NOT THROWN HER AS HIGH AND AS FAR AS SHE HAD HOPED.

I READ SOMETHING LIKE THAT IN LONDON FIELDS BY MARTIN AMIS YEARS AGO, I THINK I DID AT ANY RATE AND HAVE BEEN QUOTING IT TO STUDENTS EVER SINCE. I HOPE IT REASSURES THEM, BUT PROBABLY

THEY JUST FEEL SORRY FOR ME.

FOOD LOOKS LIKE IT WILL BE THE FIRST BATTLEFIELD. ON THE ONE SIDE ARE THE DOCTORS AND THE NUTRITIONISTS AND MOST OF MY DISINTERESTED FRIENDS. THEY ALL SAY EAT WHATEVER YOU CAN TOLERATE OVER THE NEXT SEVEN WEEKS AS LONG AS YOU KEEP YOUR WEIGHT UP.

CAKE

ICE CREAM

ON THE OTHER SIDE IS JUDE, THE INTERNET AND MANY ART WORLD PERSONALITIES.

THEY SAY SUGAR IS POISON! QUINOA, RAW VEGETABLES AND LEGUMES WILL WORK.

AVOCADO

HOMOS

JUICING KALE CARROT PARSLEY BEET APPLE

THEY SAY AVOID MEGA DOSES OF SUPLEMENT THAT CAN FEED YOUR TUMORS AS EASILY AS EASILY AS THEY CAN FIGHT THEM.

TOFU

BEHIND BOTH LURKS BOTH THE PLEASURE + PAIN PRINCIPLES. THERE IS AN ALMOST PURITANICAL ZEOL WITH WHICH SWEETS + SALTS + FATS ARE EXCISED FROM A 'HEALTHY DIET' CANCER THAT!).

ON THE OTHER HAND THERE IS
SOMETHING THAT FEELS PATRONIZING
ABOUT THE WAY THE DOCTORS + NUTRITIONISTS
TELL ME NOT TO WORRY ABOUT EATING
CRAP WHILE I'M DOING RADIATION. AS IF
I CAN'T BE TRUSTED TO KEEP MY WEIGHT
UP UNLESS I EAT LIKE A GREEDY CHILD.

I SUPPOSE FOOD IS ONE OF THE FEW
THINGS THAT ARE UNDER MY CONTROL THAT
MAY AFFECT THE OUTCOME OF THIS DISEASE
I GUESS THAT'S WHY ORGANIZED PEOPLE ARE
SERIOUS ABOUT WHAT THEY EAT AND A REALITY
DEFICIENT PERSON LIKE ME HATES TO THINK
ABOUT FOOD AT ALL...

EITHER THIS IS A GAME AND
I'M JUST BEING SPOILED FOR TWO
~~WEEKS~~ MONTHS
AND THEN I'LL RETURN
TO NORMAL AND
BE DISAPPOINTED
NOT TO
BE SPECIAL
ANYMORE.

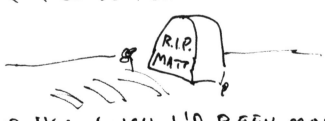

OR I'LL BE DEAD IN A YEAR.

R.I.P.
MATT

AND I'LL WISH I'D BEEN MORE
SERIOUS ABOUT THINGS. OR AT
LEAST MY FRIENDS WILL WISH THAT.

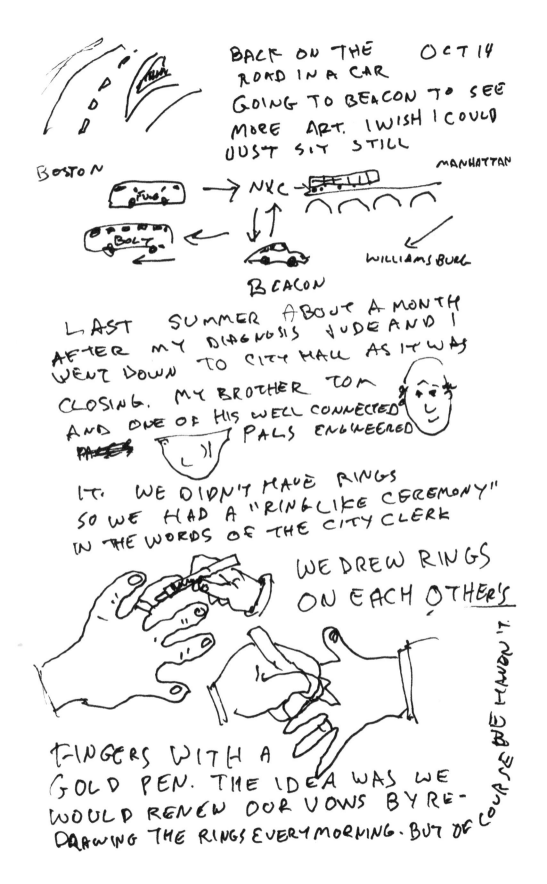

BACK ON THE OCT 14
ROAD IN A CAR
GOING TO BEACON TO SEE
MORE ART. I WISH I COULD
JUST SIT STILL

BOSTON   MANHATTAN

→ NYC →

BOLT ←

BEACON   WILLIAMSBURG

LAST SUMMER ABOUT A MONTH
AFTER MY DIAGNOSIS JUDE AND I
WENT DOWN TO CITY HALL AS IT WAS
CLOSING. MY BROTHER TOM
AND ONE OF HIS WELL CONNECTED
PALS ENGINEERED

IT. WE DIDN'T HAVE RINGS
SO WE HAD A "RING LIKE CEREMONY"
IN THE WORDS OF THE CITY CLERK

WE DREW RINGS
ON EACH OTHER'S

FINGERS WITH A
GOLD PEN. THE IDEA WAS WE
WOULD RENEW OUR VOWS BY RE-
DRAWING THE RINGS EVERY MORNING. BUT OF COURSE WE HAVEN'T.

AFTER 27 YEARS TOGETHER
I SUPPOSE IT WAS ABOUT TIME ANYWAY,
BUT IT WAS ALSO ALL ABOUT THE
INSURANCE aetna + [cross] INDEPENDENT BLUE CROSS

WE ARE LINKED BY MEDICAL
EMERGENCIES. IN 1984 I HAD JUST
MOVED TO IOWA CITY TO STUDY IN
THE GRAD SCULPTURE PROGRAM AT
THE UNIVERSITY OF IOWA. THE SCULPTURE
GRADS THERE DID ONE THING: CAST
IRON USING HOMEMADE CUPOLAS AND
RECYCLED IRON.

CUPOLA MADE
WITH OLD
GARBAGE
CANS

FORCED AIR
USING OLD
VACCUUM CLEANERS

TUB

RADIATOR

SINK

SLEDGE HAMMER
BUSTS CAST IRON INTO
CHIPS

MOLDS MADE
FROM SAND
MIXED WITH
PLASTIC POLYMER
IN HOMEMADE MULLER

SAND

SAND MIXED WITH POLYMER BINDER
THROWN OUT BY CENTRIFUGAL FORCE
YOU WERE SUPPOSED TO CATCH
THE SAND WITH A LITTLE HAND
SCOOP.

I WAS MAKING A NINE FOOT TALL FIGURE, MY FIRST LARGE SCULPTURE AND I DID NOT KNOW WHAT I WAS DOING.

I WAS MAKING THE MOLDS FOR THE SCULPTURE MUCH TOO BIG. AND SO I WAS MIXING HUNDREDS AND HUNDREDS OF POUNDS OF SAND. I WAS VERY TIRED.

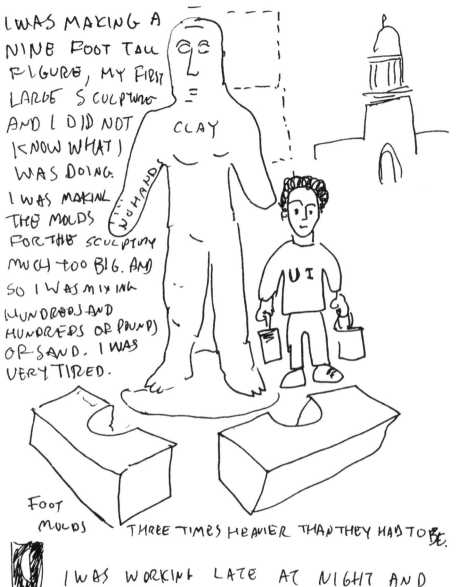

CLAY

NO HAND

FOOT MOLDS

THREE TIMES HEAVIER THAN THEY HAD TO BE.

I WAS WORKING LATE AT NIGHT AND WAS RUSHING TO FINISH BEFORE WE HAD OUR NEXT POUR. TO SAVE TIME I USED MY HAND INSTEAD OF THE SCOOP TO CATCH THE SAND. I MUST HAVE LET MY THUMB GET INSIDE THE DOOR OF THE MULLER.

THE BLADE HIT MY THUMB AND KNOCKED ME ACROSS THE ROOM

I KNEW I WAS BADLY HURT.

SOMEONE KNEW JUDE HAD A CAR. ASKED HER TO DRIVE US TO THE HOSPITAL.

SHE HAD A HUGE OLD IMPALA CONVERTIBLE.

WE FOUND THE HOSPITAL AND THEY RUSHED ME INTO THE EMERGENCY ROOM.

☒ ✓
OE

NOT CUT OFF,
CUT IN TWO

ONE OF MY FRIENDS IN THE ROOM PASSED OUT.

WHEN THE DOCTOR CUT OFF MY GLOVE MY THUMB FELL APART, THUMP! LIKE IT WAS MADE OF RUBBER.

JUDE CAME OVER AND HELD MY GOOD HAND. AS I WAS GOING INTO SHOCK I LOOKED UP AT HER AND THOUGHT,
"AT LEAST I GOT TO MEET JUDE TALLICHET"

HE'S KIND OF CUTE

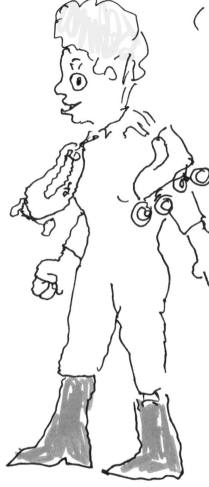

(DRAWING ON BUS FROM
NYC TO BOSTON FOR
4:30 PROTON TREATMENT)
EXCUSE THE SHAKINESS

I FIRST SAW JUDE
WHEN SHE WAS WALKING
THROUGH THE SCRAP
YARD THAT WAS THE
SCULPTURE STUDIO.
SHE WORE A SIREN
SUIT, RED COWBOY
BOOTS AND SHE HAD
A PAIR OF GOLDEN
OLD FASHIONED ROLLER
SKATES SLUNG OVER
HER SHOULDER. SHE
HAD AN ASYMMETRIC
HAIR CUT, CURLY ON TOP
SHAVED CLOSE IN THE
BACK.

I THOUGHT SHE WAS A FRESHMAN, SHE SMILED
TOO BROADLY TO BE ON THE FACULTY OR EVEN IN
GRAD SCHOOL. I THOUGHT SHE WAS THE
KIND OF BEAUTIFUL TOUGH GIRL I COULD
NEVER MEET.   IT TURNED OUT SHE WAS
                                    A PROF-
                                    FESSOR.

THANK GOD I CUT MY FINGER
IN TWO. THAT WAS PROBABLY MY
ONLY CHANCE.

JUDE HAD WORKED ON RANCHES
IN MONTANA FOR YEARS. ONCE
SHE WAS PAID FOR A YEAR IN MEAT.

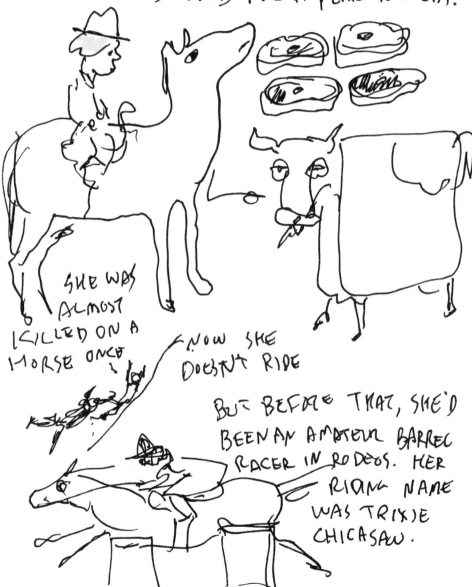

SHE WAS
ALMOST
KILLED ON A
HORSE ONCE

NOW SHE
DOESN'T RIDE

BUT BEFORE THAT, SHE'D
BEEN AN AMATEUR BARREL
RACER IN RODEOS. HER
RIDING NAME
WAS TRIXIE
CHICASAW.

TRIX IS NOW MY NAME ONLINE...

NEEDLESS TO SAY, THERE IS AN ENORMOUS COOLNESS GAP BETWEEN JUDE AND ME.

COOL

JUDE   MATT

JUDE ONCE LEFT $20,000 IN A GAS STATION BATHROOM BY MISTAKE. IT BELONGED TO A DRUG DEALER. NOTHING HAPPENED.

THERE IS A PICTURE OF JUDE COVERED IN NOTHING BUT CLAY SLIP IN AN OLD WHOLE EARTH CATALOG

JUDE WAS THE DRUMMER FOR THE BAND "THE ULTRA VULVAS!"

SHE WON MANY PRIZES AS A MARATHON RUNNER.

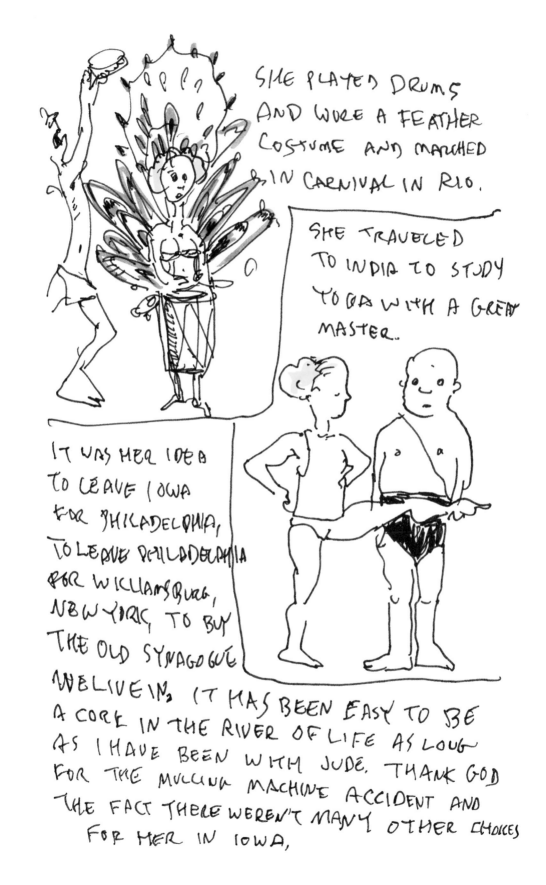

SHE PLAYED DRUMS AND WORE A FEATHER COSTUME AND MARCHED IN CARNIVAL IN RIO.

SHE TRAVELED TO INDIA TO STUDY YOGA WITH A GREAT MASTER.

IT WAS HER IDEA TO LEAVE IOWA FOR PHILADELPHIA, TO LEAVE PHILADELPHIA FOR WILLIAMSBURG, NEW YORK, TO BUY THE OLD SYNAGOGUE WE LIVE IN. IT HAS BEEN EASY TO BE A CORK IN THE RIVER OF LIFE AS LONG AS I HAVE BEEN WITH JUDE. THANK GOD FOR THE MULCHING MACHINE ACCIDENT AND THE FACT THERE WEREN'T MANY OTHER CHOICES FOR HER IN IOWA.

MUSIC IN THE PROTON CHAMBER
DAY ONE: GENERIC POP
DAY TWO: GENERIC FOLK
DAY THREE: BLUES
DAY FOUR: BAROQUE HORNS

THIS MORNING A 4:45 AM
I WOKE UP WITH USUAL
DRYNESS AND HEAD
BANGING. IN THE MIRROR
I SAW THE FIRST
IRREFUTABLE SIGNS OF
DECAY: THE BEGINNING OF A
RED NECK.

IMMEDIATELY AFTER THE RADIATION
YESTERDAY I COULD FEEL LOOSE
SKIN INSIDE MY JAW, LIKE FROM
A HOT PIZZA CHEESE BURN.

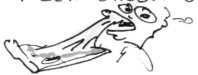

BROTHER JOSH ASKED THE SENSIBLE
QUESTION: "DOES THAT MEAN THE
PROTONS ARE GOING THROUGH THE
JAW TO THE TUMOR IN THE TONGUE,
WHICH IS NOT WHAT WE COUNTED ON.

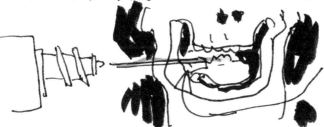

CHEESEY
PIZZA
SKIN EFFECT

IT BOTHERS ME THAT I DON'T ASK THE RIGHT QUESTIONS, THAT I HOPE FOR THE BEST. THIS THE THIRD PERSONA I AM JUGGLING AS THE TREATMENT GOES FORWARD.

①

BIG BABY (SORRY, CHARLES)

WHINEY, QUICK TO TAKE OFFENSE, UNABLE TO TOLERATE COMPLEXITY, SEEN MOSTLY BY JUDE.

②

JOE COOL

FUNNY, IRREVERENT. BRAVE IN A DISARMINGLY SELF - DEPRICATING WAY.

WHAT I TRY TO CONVEY TO FRIENDS + FAMILY.

3. MR. PASSIVE. THE NEWEST CHARACTER. EATS, SLEEPS, WATCHES THINGS. HOPES FOR THE BEST.

ONE OTHER MILESTONE YESTERDAY, MY FIRST CHANCE TO PLAY WHAT MAY BE YET ANOTHER CHARACTER, THE <u>WIZENED OLD CANCER GUY</u>.

A VERY TALL, ELEGANT COUPLE WAS WAITING FOR THE WOMAN'S FIRST RADIATION TREATMENT.

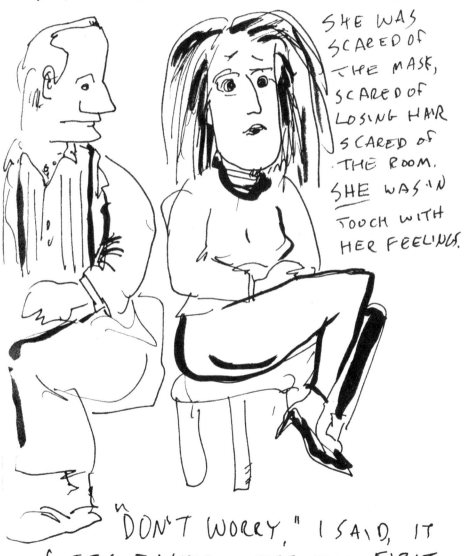

SHE WAS SCARED OF THE MASK, SCARED OF LOSING HAIR SCARED OF THE ROOM. SHE WAS <u>IN</u> TOUCH WITH HER FEELINGS.

"DON'T WORRY," I SAID, IT GETS EASIER AFTER THE FIRST TREATMENT." I HAVE NO IDEA IF THIS IS TRUE.

THE NUTRITIONIST MET ME TODAY
AND PREPARED ME FOR THE FUTURE:
BOWLS OF YOGURT AND SOUP. NUT
BUTTER MIXED WITH ENSURE. SHE
FALLS MORE ON THE NATURAL SIDE
BUT ALSO WANTS CALORIES, HYDRATION
AND PROTIENS UBER ALLES.

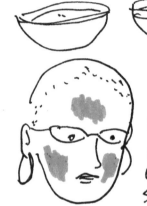

SHE HAD
VERY SHORT
HAIR AND BIG   OR IT'S THE
EARRINGS. TOWARDS   TUBE
THE END
OF THE SESSION SHE TOLD ME
SHE WAS IN TREATMENT TOO.
IT WAS VERY CUTE AND TOUCHING.

THIS IS THE THIRD PERSON FROM THE
MEDICAL SIDE WHO HAS MENTIONED
THEIR OWN CANCER HISTORY. IT'S

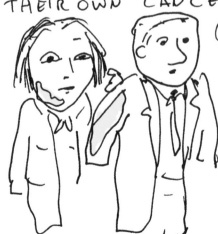

GOOD TO HEAR THEIR
STORIES. THE WORLD
IS (TEMPORARILY?)
BREAKING INTO THOSE
WHO HAVE (HAD)
CANCER AND THOSE
WHO HAVEN'T (YET).

MUSIC YESTERDAY THE ~~BEATLES~~ IN BEATLES HONOR OF MY SHIRT

BUT AFTER 10 MINUTES THEY SWITCHED TO MORE GENERIC POP

HEY JUDE 1968

EFFECT THEY HAD ON MY FRIEND BILL, WHO WENT ON AN OCCASIONALLY INAPPROPRIATE TALKING JAG

LAST NIGHT I TOOK MY FIRST TWO ANTI-NAUSEA PILLS* THEY DIDN'T HAVE THE

OR JOHN, WHO PAINTED UP A STORM

OR TONI WHO RAN ALL OVER THE CITY AND WROTE A PLAY.

IT DID, HOWEVER, HAVE ANOTHER ODD EFFECT ON ME.

THE MOST DISTURBING EFFECT

HOWEVER, IS THE INCREASING FOGGINESS OF MY BRAIN. YESTERDAY I WAS WRITING TO A FRIEND AND COULDN'T REMEMBER AN OBSCURE LANGUAGE'S NAME. I KNEW IT WAS USED IN A MOVIE ABOUT JESUS CHRIST, BUT I COULDN'T REMEMBER THE NAME OF THE MOVIE. I KNEW THE MOVIE WAS MADE

* FOR THE CHEMOTHERAPY

BY A FAMOUS CONTROVERSIAL MOVIE STAR, BUT I COULDN'T REMEMBER HIS NAME. I DID REMEMBER ROADWARRIOR FINALLY, WHICH LED TO MADMAX, WHICH LED TO MEL GIBSON, WHICH LED TO THE PASSION OF THE CHRIST, WHICH LED FINALLY, TO ARAMAIC, THOUGH THAT MIGHT ACTUALLY NOT BE THE RIGHT LANGUAGE IN THE FIRST PLACE.

WIKIPEDIA

LECTURE AT THE HARVARD COOP BY ARAMAIC SPEAKER COULD BE INTERESTING

ON THE OTHER HAND MNEMONIC DEVICE WISE, NUMBERS SEEM TO BE STAYING PUT.
THE FIRST DAY WE PARKED IN STALL 406.
TED WILLIAMS BATTING AVERAGE IN 1941. THE LAST 400 HITTER.

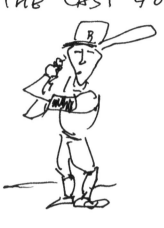

THE NEXT DAY WE PARKED IN 388 ROD CAREW'S HIGHEST AVERAGE.

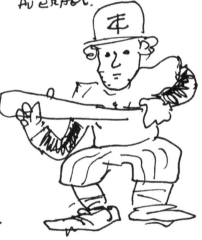

THE NEXT DAY ~~NIGHT~~ WAS 231 I GOT NOTHING FOR THAT, SO IT STUCK BECAUSE OF THAT.

NO ONE HIT 231 HOME RUNS EXACTLY BUT ROB DEER HIT 230.

TODAY WAS 51, CECIL FIELDER'S, PRINCE'S DAD, HIGH WATER MARK.

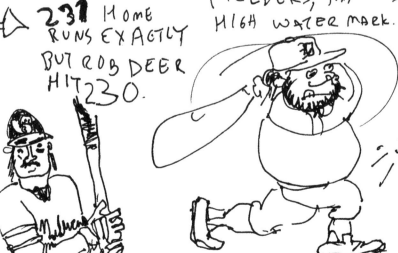

SITTING IN INFUSION ROOM GETTING MY FIRST CHEMO. ODD THEY USE THE SAME WORDS TO DESCRIBE TEA BREWING.

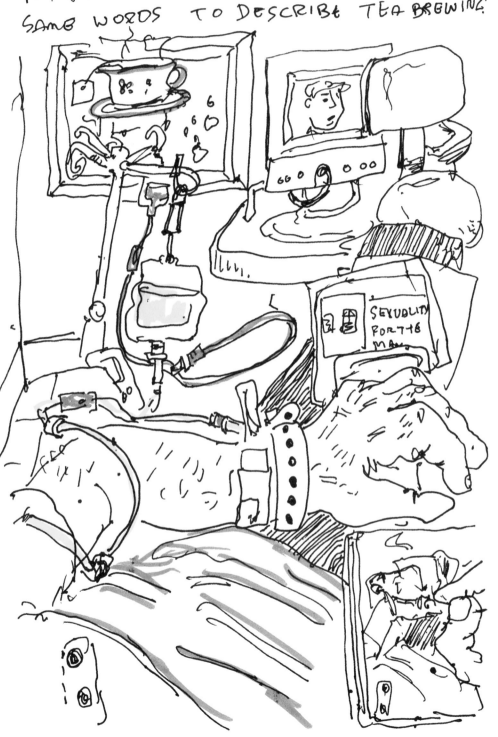

DAY 7 ⅕ DONE [OCT 18

20%

AM MUSIC REPORT I'M BRINGING IN A RAY CHARLES CD

YESTERDAY IN THE MIDDLE OF THE 3:45 MINUTE CHEMO SESSION THE FRIENDLY CHATTY NURSE SUPPLYING THE DRUGS ALLOWED AS HOW THEY WERE HOPING TO GIVE ME "TWO GOOD YEARS" WHILE THE SEARCH WENT ON FOR THE CURRENTLY UNCURABLE CANCER IN MY LUNGS. THIS WAS THE FIRST TIME THAT ANYONE ON THE MEDICAL SIDE VOLUNTARILY GAVE UP A NUMBER OF YEARS LEFT. AND IT ALMOST SLID BY WITHOUT NOTICE. DID I MISHEAR? WAS THIS AN INFORMATION LEAK? A YANK ON THE CURTAIN THAT I HAVE PULLED AROUND ME?

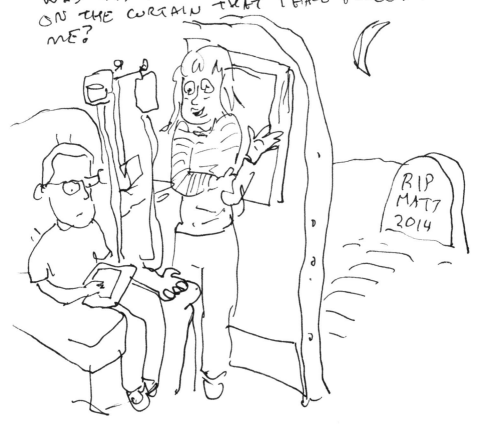

JOSH AND FAMILY ARRIVED AT AROUND
MIDNIGHT AFTER A SIX HOUR FLIGHT FROM
CALIFORNIA. NINA, JOSH'S WIFE HAD A
MIGRAINE AND STAYED IN A HOTEL. JOSH
CAME OVER WITH HIS KIDS ELI AND ABE.
ALL THINGS CONSIDERED THEY WERE
IN GREAT SHAPE AFTER SUCH A LONG
FLIGHT, BUT ABE WAS A BIT OBSESSED
WITH PLAYING WITH HIS IPAD, WHICH
HAD BEEN PACKED AWAY. JOSH IS THE
MOST PATIENT AND THOUGHTFUL DAD AND
KEPT UP A REASONABLE CONVERSATION WITH
THE DETERMINED ABE FOR AT LEAST HALF
AN HOUR, WHILE I SLOWLY TURNED INTO <u>A
GRUMPY OLD MAN</u>. FINALLY I SAID "ABE!"
AND JOSH SAID "UNCLE MATT IS UPSET!"
AND ELI SAID "WHY IS UNCLE MATT UPSET?"
AND JOSH SAID "BECAUSE OF ABE" AND ELI
SAID "OH." AND POOR ABE QUICKLY ABANDONED
HIS QUEST. SO THAT'S PERSONA NUMBER 5

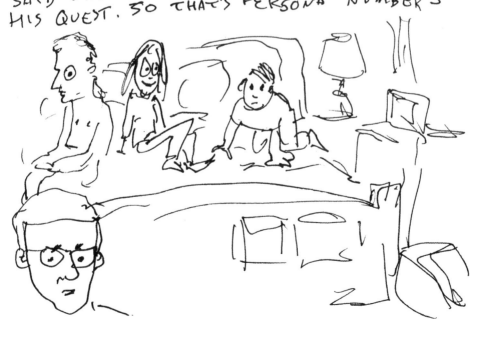

JOSH'S DIAGRAM EXPLAINING SOME RECENT RESEARCH THAT INDICATES ACC MAY COME ABOUT WHEN ~~THE~~ ~~~~ CHROMOSOME 6 ATTACHES TO THE CHROMOSOME 9 SLOT DURING GENE SPLITING.

translate

promoter   gene protein sequence

gene protein product

WHEN THE WRONG PROMOTER GETS AHOLD OF THIS PROTIEN THINGS GO WRONG.

MYB 6 NFIB 9

THE RESEARCH THAT MAY HELP FIGHT THE LUNG METASTESES WOULD SPRESS THE MYB PROTIEN THAT GOES WILD WHEN THIS MIS- MATCH OCCURS. MOST PEOPLES' MISMATCHTES GO NOWHERE.
BUT NOT ACC PEOPLE

3:15 THURSDAY

ETHAN CASCIO RADIATION TEST PROGRAM MANAGER LECTURE ON PROTON THERAPY HISTORY AND TECHNIQUE

BRAGG PEAK

PERCENTAL EFFECT

PEAK PATTERN OF PROTON PENETRPT

DEPTH →

SPINNER THAT THOWS PROTONS

DOSE

PHOTONS
PROTON
IDEAL

STEEP FALL OFF OF PROTONS IS WHY THEY ARE BETTER THAN PHOTONS.

PHOTON
PROTON

DEPTH

NORMAL TARGET   NORMAL
SURFACE DIE   SOAP

ETHAN PASSES OUT SAMPLES.

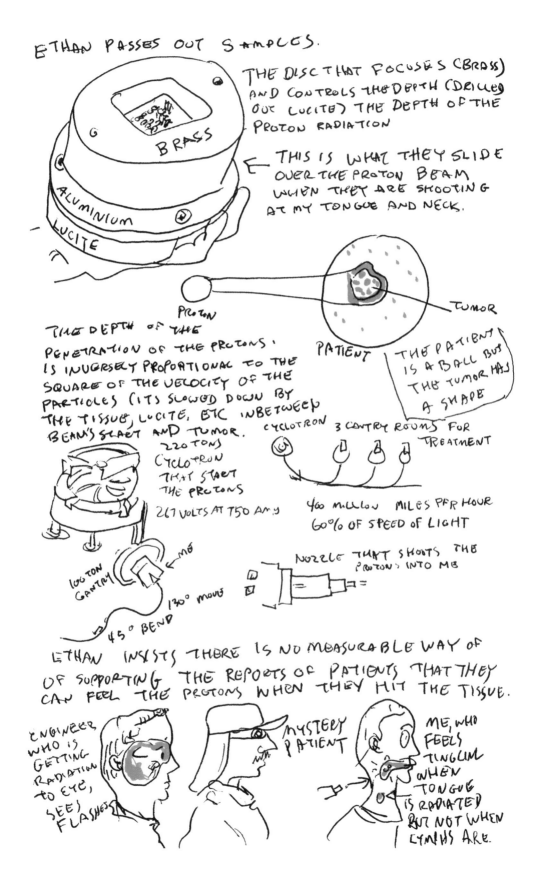

THE DISC THAT FOCUSES (BRASS) AND CONTROLS THE DEPTH (DRILLED OUT LUCITE) THE DEPTH OF THE PROTON RADIATION

BRASS

ALUMINIUM

LUCITE

THIS IS WHAT THEY SLIDE OVER THE PROTON BEAM WHEN THEY ARE SHOOTING AT MY TONGUE AND NECK.

PROTON

PATIENT

TUMOR

THE PATIENT IS A BALL BUT THE TUMOR HAS A SHAPE

THE DEPTH OF THE PENETRATION OF THE PROTONS IS INVERSELY PROPORTIONAL TO THE SQUARE OF THE VELOCITY OF THE PARTICLES (ITS SLOWED DOWN BY THE TISSUE, LUCITE, ETC INBETWEEN BEAM'S START AND TUMOR.

CYCLOTRON

3 GANTRY ROOMS FOR TREATMENT

220 TONS CYCLOTRON THAT START THE PROTONS

267 VOLTS AT 750 AMP

460 MILLION MILES PER HOUR 60% OF SPEED OF LIGHT

100 TON GANTRY

M8

45° BEND

130° MOVES

NOZZLE THAT SHOOTS THE PROTONS INTO M8

ETHAN INSISTS THERE IS NO MEASURABLE WAY OF OF SUPPORTING THE REPORTS OF PATIENTS THAT THEY CAN FEEL THE PROTONS WHEN THEY HIT THE TISSUE.

ENGINEER WHO IS GETTING RADIATION TO EYE, SEES FLASHES

MYSTERY PATIENT

ME, WHO FEELS TINGLING WHEN TONGUE IS RADIATED BUT NOT WHEN LYMPHS ARE.

BACH
CELLO SOLO

STALL
258

LAST NIGHT AS I WAS DRIVING JOSH AND ABE BACK TO THE APARTMENT ABE ASKED,

ARE YOU GOING TO BE THE FIRST UNCLE TO DIE

BECAUSE YOU'RE SICK?

WELL, THAT'S CERTAINLY MY PLAN!

I DIDN'T HAVE A GOOD ANSWER SO I WENT RIGHT FOR A JOKE.
WHY DID I SAY THAT TO A LITTLE KID? WAS I TRYING TO BE LIGHT HEARTED? WAS I BEING MEAN? WAS I TORTURING MYSELF? WHY WOULD THAT EVEN OCCUR TO ANYBODY TO SAY? IT MAKES NO SENSE AT ALL.

ASKED FOR A CHEST SCAN DESPITE DOCTORS' OBJECTIONS. MAYBE MORE DATA WILL HELP, MAYBE NOT
*

* THE QUESTION: ARE THE LUNG TUMORS GROWING (FAST)?

FOOD IS ALMOST TASTELESS ALREADY BUT I CONTINUE TO EAT ENORMOUS AMOUNTS. I WAS UP SEVEN POUNDS AT THIS MORNING'S WEIGH IN, BUT

THAT'S BECAUSE THINGS HAVE STOPPED
FLOWING NICELY IN ONE END AND
OUT THE OTHER. NOTHING YET THAT
SCIENCE, FOLK MEDICINE AND WILL POWER
CAN'T OVERCOME.

THIS AFTERNOON MY FRIEND CAROLINE
CALLED ABOUT A SHOW SHE IS ORGANIZING.
SHE HAS ASKED ME TO PARTICIPATE AND
WANTS TO KNOW WHEN I WOULD WANT
TO HAVE THE SHOW HAPPEN. IN LIGHT
OF MY CONDITION I GET SOME SAY.
ONE OF THE OTHER ARTISTS, WARD,
SAYS HE COULD BE READY WITH HIS
PART OF THE SHOW IN TEN MONTHS

IS THAT ENOUGH TIME? TOO MUCH? TOO LITTLE?

AND I SAY

THAT SOUND) OKAY

YOU DON'T WANT MORE TIME?

NO, I THINK THAT MIGHT NOT BE A GOOD IDEA. I DON'T THINK I SHOULD ORDER GREEN BANANAS THESE DAYS.

WHY DID I SAY THAT? WAS I STILL AFFECTED BY ABE'S QUESTION? OR AM I JUST TURNING INTO A JERK?

THERE IS A BEAUTIFUL PATIO GARDEN ON THE EIGHTH FLOOR OF THE HOSPITAL BUILDING. IT'S ALREADY FADING FROM MEMORY. BYE.

THERE WAS SOME KIND OF CUPOLA ROOFTOP NEARBY.

YOU CAN SEE THE BRIDGE ACROSS

THE CHARLES RIVER TO CAMBRIDGE.

THERE WERE A LOT OF URNS.

JOSH TALKS TO OLD FRIEND WHO IS ON STAFF AT MGH.

HE DISCUSSES THE COGNITIVE THEORY OF THE BRAIN. OUR SIMPLE LIZARD BRAINS NEED POSITIVE REINFORCEMENT TO WORK AT PEAK EFFECTIVENESS.

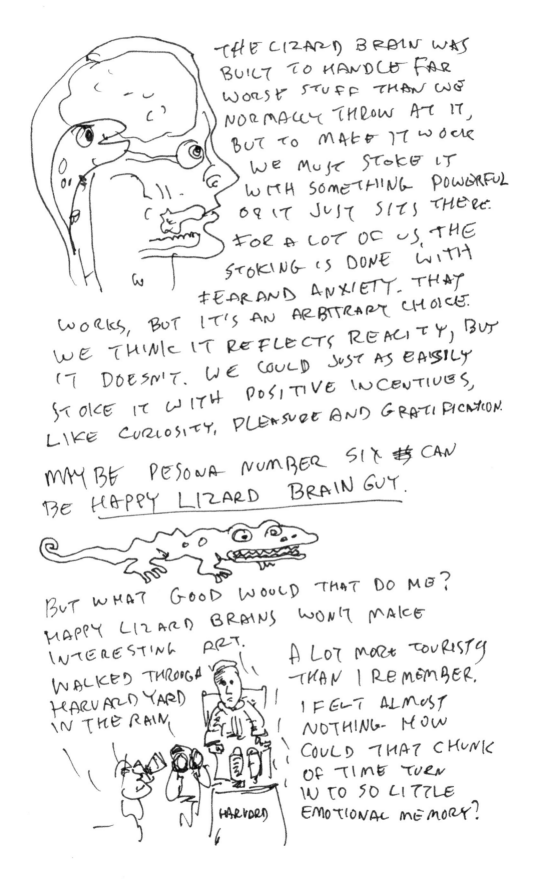

THE LIZARD BRAIN WAS BUILT TO HANDLE FAR WORSE STUFF THAN WE NORMALLY THROW AT IT, BUT TO MAKE IT WORK WE MUST STOKE IT WITH SOMETHING POWERFUL OR IT JUST SITS THERE. FOR A LOT OF US, THE STOKING IS DONE WITH FEAR AND ANXIETY. THAT

WORKS, BUT IT'S AN ARBITRARY CHOICE. WE THINK IT REFLECTS REALITY, BUT IT DOESN'T. WE COULD JUST AS EASILY STOKE IT WITH POSITIVE INCENTIVES, LIKE CURIOSITY, PLEASURE AND GRATIFICATION.

MAYBE PESONA NUMBER SIX # CAN BE HAPPY LIZARD BRAIN GUY.

BUT WHAT GOOD WOULD THAT DO ME? HAPPY LIZARD BRAINS WON'T MAKE INTERESTING ART.

WALKED THROUGH HARVARD YARD IN THE RAIN,

A LOT MORE TOURISTY THAN I REMEMBER. I FELT ALMOST NOTHING. HOW COULD THAT CHUNK OF TIME TURN INTO SO LITTLE EMOTIONAL MEMORY?

HARVARD

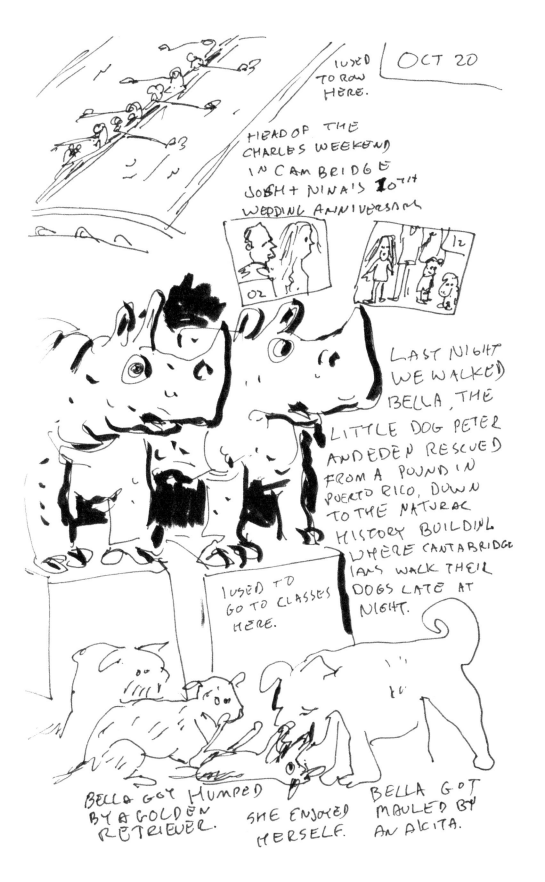

I USED TO ROW HERE.

OCT 20

HEAD OF THE CHARLES WEEKEND IN CAMBRIDGE JOSH + NINA'S 10TH WEDDING ANNIVERSARY

02

12

LAST NIGHT WE WALKED BELLA, THE LITTLE DOG PETER AND EDEN RESCUED FROM A POUND IN PUERTO RICO, DOWN TO THE NATURAL HISTORY BUILDING WHERE CANTABRIDGEIANS WALK THEIR DOGS LATE AT NIGHT.

I USED TO GO TO CLASSES HERE.

BELLA GOT HUMPED BY A GOLDEN RETRIEVER.

SHE ENJOYED HERSELF.

BELLA GOT MAULED BY AN AKITA.

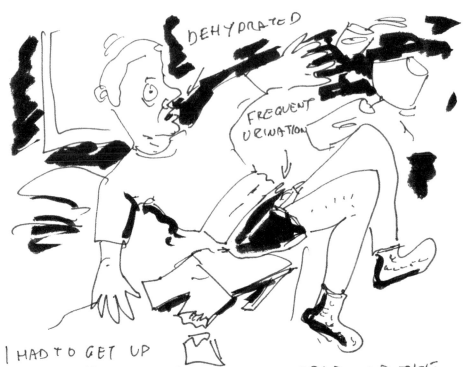

I HAD TO GET UP
FOUR OR FIVE TIMES IN THE MIDDLE OF THE
NIGHT. ONCE I MISSED THE BED COMING BACK
AND SAT DOWN HARD ON A LITTLE STOOL, BREAKING
IT. IT WAS MY FIRST CONFUSED SICK OLD
MAN MOVE, SO FAR.

THE COMPETITIVE SIDE OF ME AT
LEAST WANTS TO HANDLE THIS AS
SMOOTHLY AS POSSIBLE. I WANT TO
GAIN WEIGHT, NOT LOSE WEIGHT FOR
AS LONG AS POSSIBLE. I WANT TO KEEP
MY ACT TOGETHER JUST TO PROVE I
CAN. PART JOE COOL PART BIG JERK

CANCER SCHMANCER!

BRING IT ON.

IMPRESSIVE

BUT NOTHING I CAN DO FOR SHEER MACHISMO WILL MATCH MY OLD PROFESSOR JULIUS SCHMIDT. (HE WAS ALMOST 70 AT THE TIME) 1985 DURING AN IRON POUR HE DIPPED A WET SKIMMER INTO A LADLE OF MOLTEN IRON. IT BLEW UP IN HIS FACE

KABOOM!

HIS FACE BURNED BY IRON IN A DOZEN PLACES, HE DROVE HIMSELF TO THE HOSPITAL.

WHEN WE VISITED HIM IN THE HOSPITAL HE WAS IN INTENSIVE CARE.

EVERYONE ELSE IN THE BURN UNIT WAS MISSING HANDS OR FEET OR PART OF THEIR FACE.

HE CAME BACK TO CLASS THE NEXT DAY, LOOKING LIKE A MONSTER. THEY SAID HE WOULD BE SCARRED FOR LIFE. BUT HE SHAVED THE BURNED SKIN OFF HIS FACE WITH A RAZOR EVERY DAY FOR A WEEK AND CAME BACK LOOKING YOUNGER THAN EVER.

THE DOCTORS WERE AMAZED!

HE SAID WITH GREAT SATISFACTION.

WHAT DID I LEARN FROM THAT? WHAT MAKES A GOOD TEACHER. JULIUS TAUGHT PURELY BY POWER OF WILL. ONCE HE CUT UP THE CARPET IN HIS OFFICE TO GIVE ME MATERIAL FOR A MOLD. I THINK HE WAS TEACHING ABOUT COMMITMENT

BUT SHOULD TEACHING ENCOURAGE ALL THE TIME, OR SHOULD IT DISCOURAGE SOMETIMES? I ASKED MY STUDENTS TO WRITE ME WITH THEIR BEST LEARNING STORIES. ONE WOMAN WROTE ABOUT A MASTER CLASS SHE PARTICIPATED IN AT A CONSERVATORY. THE TEACHER WAS A FAMOUS CELLIST REKNOWNED FOR HIS LACK OF COMPASSION.

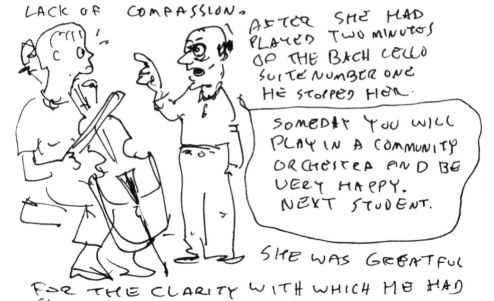

AFTER SHE HAD PLAYED TWO MINUTES OF THE BACH CELLO SUITE NUMBER ONE HE STOPPED HER.

SOMEDAY YOU WILL PLAY IN A COMMUNITY ORCHESTRA AND BE VERY HAPPY. NEXT STUDENT.

SHE WAS GREATFUL FOR THE CLARITY WITH WHICH HE HAD SIZED UP HER INTERESTS AND ABILITIES. IT SEEMED TO LIBERATE HER. THAT SCARES ME.

SECOND DAY OFF. TONGUE | OCT 21
STARTING TO GO DOWNHILL. FOOD IS
TASTELESS BUT STILL I EAT AND EAT
AND EAT. I AM GETTING FAT. LAST
NIGHT WAS JOSH AND NINA'S 10th
ANNIVERSARY. WE WENT TO ONE OF HIS
FRIEND'S BEAUTIFUL HOMES (THE BEAUTIFUL
HOME OF ONE OF HIS FRIENDS) AND HAD A
WONDERFUL MEAL.

GREEN SALAD

CHERRY TOMATOES AND MOZZARELLA

LAGAGNA

SAUTED CHICKEN BREASTS

CHEESES

ASPARAGUS WITH ASPARAGUS FORK

WINE

CHAMPAGNE

BRUT

HAPPY ANNIVERSARY

AN AMAZING MEAL. I THINK I ATE
TWICE AS MUCH AS ANYONE. YET I
COULD NOT TASTE ANYTHING AND MY
TONGUE WAS ON FIRE. BUT I KEPT
EATING. I SAID IT WAS FOR FOR THE
PROTEIN AND THE CALORIES BUT I THINK
IT IS MORE FEAR
THAN ANYTHING
ELSE.

JUDE (AND FLEURRY) ARE HERE
FOR A WEEK. ITS GOOD TO
HAVE MOST OF THE PACK TOGETHER.

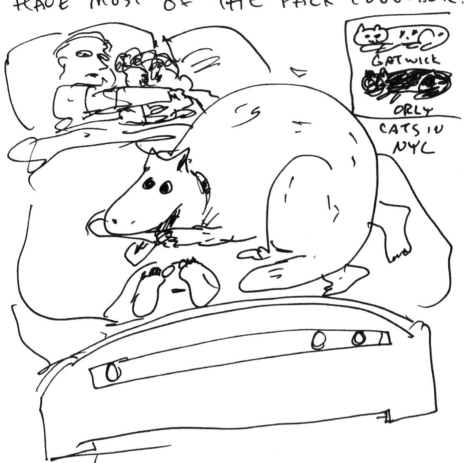

GATWICK

ORLY

CATS IN NYC

THE DOG IS A BIG PRESENCE. WALK
THE DOG, FEED THE DOG, PICKUP AFTER
THE DOG. KEEP THE DOG FROM KILLING
SQUIRRELS. ANTICIPATE DOG-DOG ENCOUNTERS.
CALCULATE POTENTIAL DOG-KID MAYHEM.

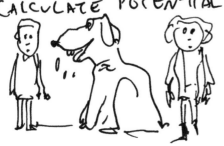

IS THIS HEALTHY?
SHOULD DOG
BE IN
BETTER
PERSPEC-
TIVE?

THIS MORNING ANOTHER TRIP TO ANOTHER
BEAUTIFUL HOME AND MORE BEAUTIFUL
FOOD THAT I COULD NOT TASTE BUT
COULD NOT STOP EATING.

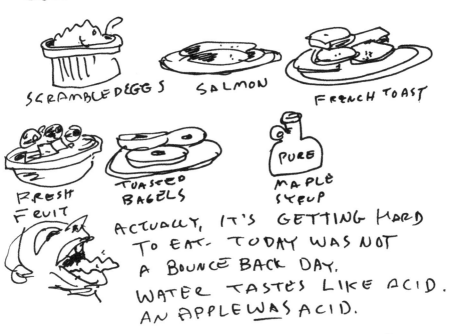

SCRAMBLED EGGS   SALMON   FRENCH TOAST

FRESH FRUIT   TOASTED BAGELS   PURE MAPLE SYRUP

ACTUALLY, IT'S GETTING HARD
TO EAT. TODAY WAS NOT
A BOUNCE BACK DAY.
WATER TASTES LIKE ACID.
AN APPLE WAS ACID.

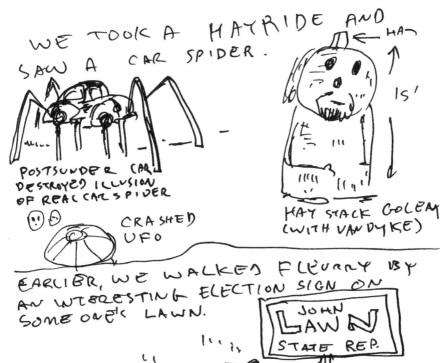

WE TOOK A HAYRIDE AND
SAW A CAR SPIDER.

← HAT

15'

POSTSUNDER CAR
DESTROYED ILLUSION
OF REAL CAR SPIDER

CRASHED UFO

HAY STACK GOLEM
(WITH VAN DYKE)

EARLIER, WE WALKED FLEURRY BY
AN INTERESTING ELECTION SIGN ON
SOME ONE'S LAWN.

JOHN
LAWN
STATE REP.

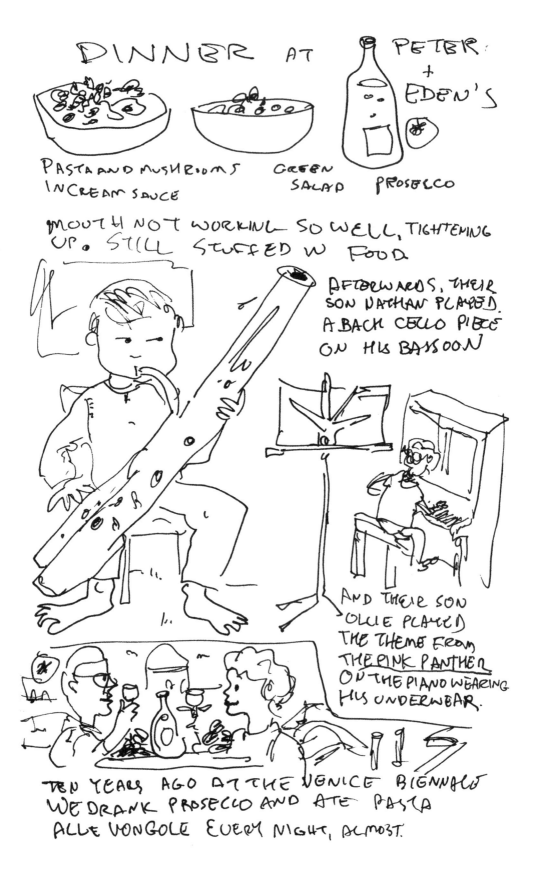

DINNER AT PETER + EDEN'S

PASTA AND MUSHROOMS
IN CREAM SAUCE

GREEN SALAD

PROSECCO

MOUTH NOT WORKING SO WELL, TIGHTENING UP. STILL STUFFED W FOOD

AFTERWARDS, THEIR SON NATHAN PLAYED A BACH CELLO PIECE ON HIS BASSOON

AND THEIR SON OLLIE PLAYED THE THEME FROM THE PINK PANTHER ON THE PIANO WEARING HIS UNDERWEAR.

TEN YEARS AGO AT THE VENICE BIENNALE WE DRANK PROSECCO AND ATE PASTA ALLE VONGOLE EVERY NIGHT, ALMOST.

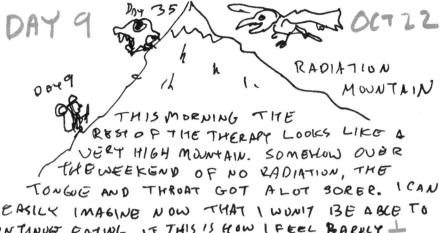

DAY 9   Day 35   OCT 22

RADIATION MOUNTAIN

Day 9

THIS MORNING THE REST OF THE THERAPY LOOKS LIKE A VERY HIGH MOUNTAIN. SOMEHOW OVER THE WEEKEND OF NO RADIATION, THE TONGUE AND THROAT GOT A LOT SORER. I CAN EASILY IMAGINE NOW THAT I WON'T BE ABLE TO CONTINUE EATING IF THIS IS HOW I FEEL BARELY $\frac{1}{4}$ OF THE WAY THROUGH.

COFFEE TOO HOT TO DRINK BLACK.
ONE COOKIE WAS LIKE EATING SHARP GRAVEL.

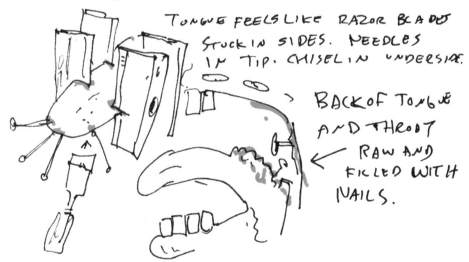

TONGUE FEELS LIKE RAZOR BLADES STUCK IN SIDES. NEEDLES IN TIP. CHISEL IN UNDERSIDE.

BACK OF TONGUE AND THROAT RAW AND FILLED WITH NAILS.

I DIDN'T MEAN TO DWELL ON THE DAY TO DAY EXPERIENCE OF EATING AND WORRYING AND MONITORING PAIN + FEAR. I THOUGHT LARGER REVELATIONS ABOUT LIFE AND DEATH WOULD BECOME APPARENT TO ME, BUT NOT SO MUCH. I'M TURNING MORE FERAL THAN PHILOSOPHICAL AS THIS WEARS ON. ONCE AGAIN, NO FREE PASS TO ENLIGHTENMENT.

| MORE PAIN | to | MORE WISDOM |

FOR THE FIRST TIME SINCE THE FIRST
SESSION THE RADIATION WAS AN ORDEAL.
THE THICK PHLEGM BEGAN TO COLLECT IN
THE   BACK OF MY THROAT.
                             THEN MY NOSE BEGAN
                             TO RUN AND MY EYES
                             TEARED UP. I HAD
                             TO STRUGGLE TO
                             SWALLOW AND THAT
                             MADE ONE OF MY
                             CLAMPS POP LOOSE
RIGHT BEFORE THEY BEGAN IRRADIATION.
NO ONE SAID ANYTHING SO I STAYED AS STILL
AS I COULD, SORT OF LIKE THE GUY WHO
HOLDS THE CARD UP FOR THE SHARPSHOOTER.

IT FELT LIKE I IMAGINE WATERBOARDING
FEELS LIKE. CORRECTION: THAT IS WHAT
JUDE SAID IT SOUNDED LIKE. NOW I HAVE
TO DEAL WITH THE IDEA THAT IT'S LIKE
WATERBOARDING FOR THE REST OF THE THERAPY.

AT LUNCH I COULD NOT
FINISH A PLATE OF MACARONI
AND CHEESE AND MASHED
POTATOES. MY THROAT HURT
TOO MUCH. THIS IS GETTING
SERIOUS.

IT'S ALSO NOW ON THE TABLE TO TAKE ATIVAN DURING TREATMENT. APPARENTLY THEY WORRY MY CHOKING UNDER THE MASK WAS A PANIC ATTACK. SO NOW I AM GOING TO START DRUGGING MYSELF?

THE BIG PROBLEM IS THE THICK PHLEGM THAT IS COATING MY MOUTH AND ~~THROAT~~ THROAT. MY SPEECH IS BECOMING AFFECTED.

THIS MORNING WE WALKED FLEURRY TO A FIELD WHERE SHE PLAYED WITH WITH A SMALL DOG. I ASKED THE DOG'S OWNER ABOUT LOCAL LEASH LAWS AND SHE COULDN'T UNDERSTAND ME.

SSLEESCH SSLAWSSS?

WHA?

THIS AFTERNOON I TRIED TO GIVE MY MOTHER THE ADDRESS OF THE HOSPITAL AND I FINALLY HAD TO GIVE THE PHONE TO JUDE.

STHIRTYSS FRUIT STREET

NO, FRUIT! FRUIT

NO, FRUIT, LIKE APPLES

FORGET IT

31ST STREET?

FORT STREET?

APPLE STREET

FORT STREET?

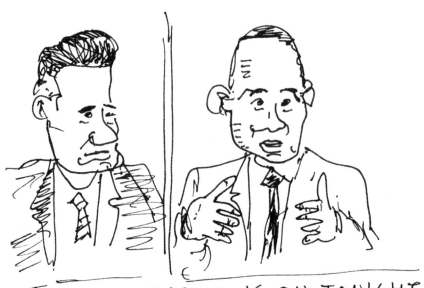

THE LAST DEBATE IS ON TONIGHT
I CAN'T SAY I HAVE EXACTLY THE SAME
PATIENCE FOR ALL THEIR TALKING POINTS.

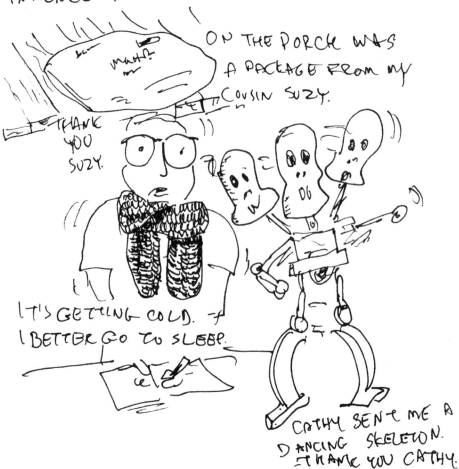

ON THE PORCH WAS A PACKAGE FROM MY COUSIN SUZY.

THANK YOU SUZY.

IT'S GETTING COLD. I BETTER GO TO SLEEP.

CATHY SENT ME A DANCING SKELETON. THANK YOU CATHY.

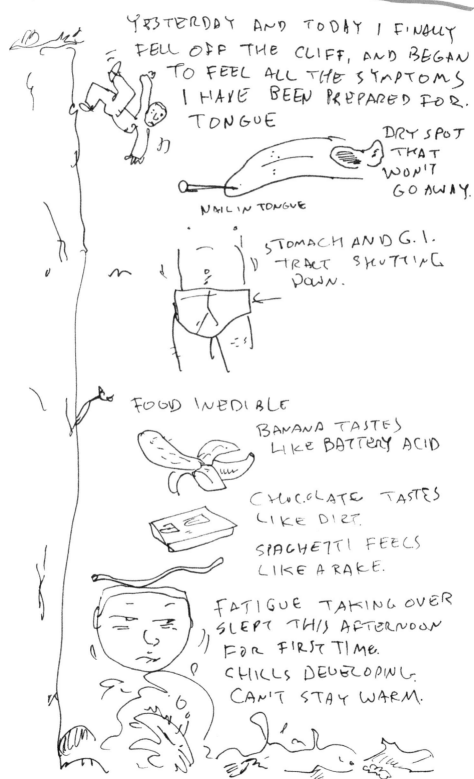

YESTERDAY AND TODAY I FINALLY FELL OFF THE CLIFF, AND BEGAN TO FEEL ALL THE SYMPTOMS I HAVE BEEN PREPARED FOR.
TONGUE

DRY SPOT THAT WON'T GO AWAY.

NAIL IN TONGUE

STOMACH AND G.I. TRACT SHUTTING DOWN.

FOOD INEDIBLE

BANANA TASTES LIKE BATTERY ACID

CHOCOLATE TASTES LIKE DIRT.

SPAGHETTI FEELS LIKE A RAKE.

FATIGUE TAKING OVER SLEPT THIS AFTERNOON FOR FIRST TIME. CHILLS DEVELOPING. CAN'T STAY WARM.

LAST NIGHT JOSH TOLD A FAMILIAR
STORY TO OUR FRIENDS. HOW MY BROTHER
BERT ~~HAD~~ AND I HAD TEASED HIM SO
MERCILESSLY ONE DAY WHEN WE WERE
KIDS AND HE WAS TRYING TO MAKE AND
RECORD HIS OWN OPERA THAT HE HAD
BURST INTO TEARS.

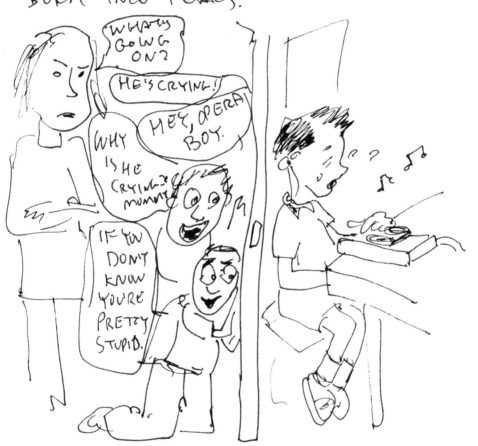

JOSH WAS TRYING TO RECORD AN OPERA
ON AN OLD TAPE TO TAPE RECORDER. WE
FELT THREATENED I GUESS BY HIS SERIOUSNESS
AND AMBITION. OUR MOTHER TRIED TO
PROTECT HIM FROM US BUT I GUESS HE WAS
DEEPLY SCARRED. HE TELLS THIS STORY A LOT.

SO NOW I'M THINKING AFTER WE GET THROUGH THE FIRST 34 DAYS OF RADIATION THE TECHNICIANS ALLOW JOSH TO APPLY THE LAST DAY'S DOSE. HE LEANS OVER AND SAYS,

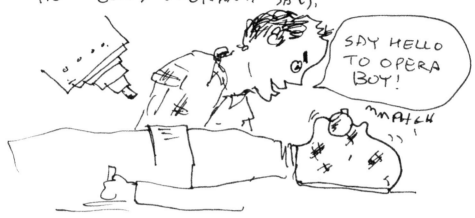

SAY HELLO TO OPERA BOY!

MMAHCH

I WENT BACK UP TO THE HEALING GARDEN AFTER THERAPY. I FELT PRETTY WIPED OUT.

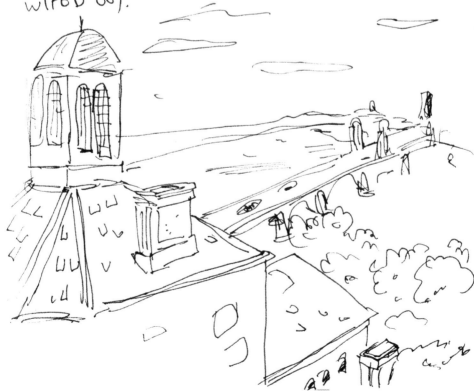

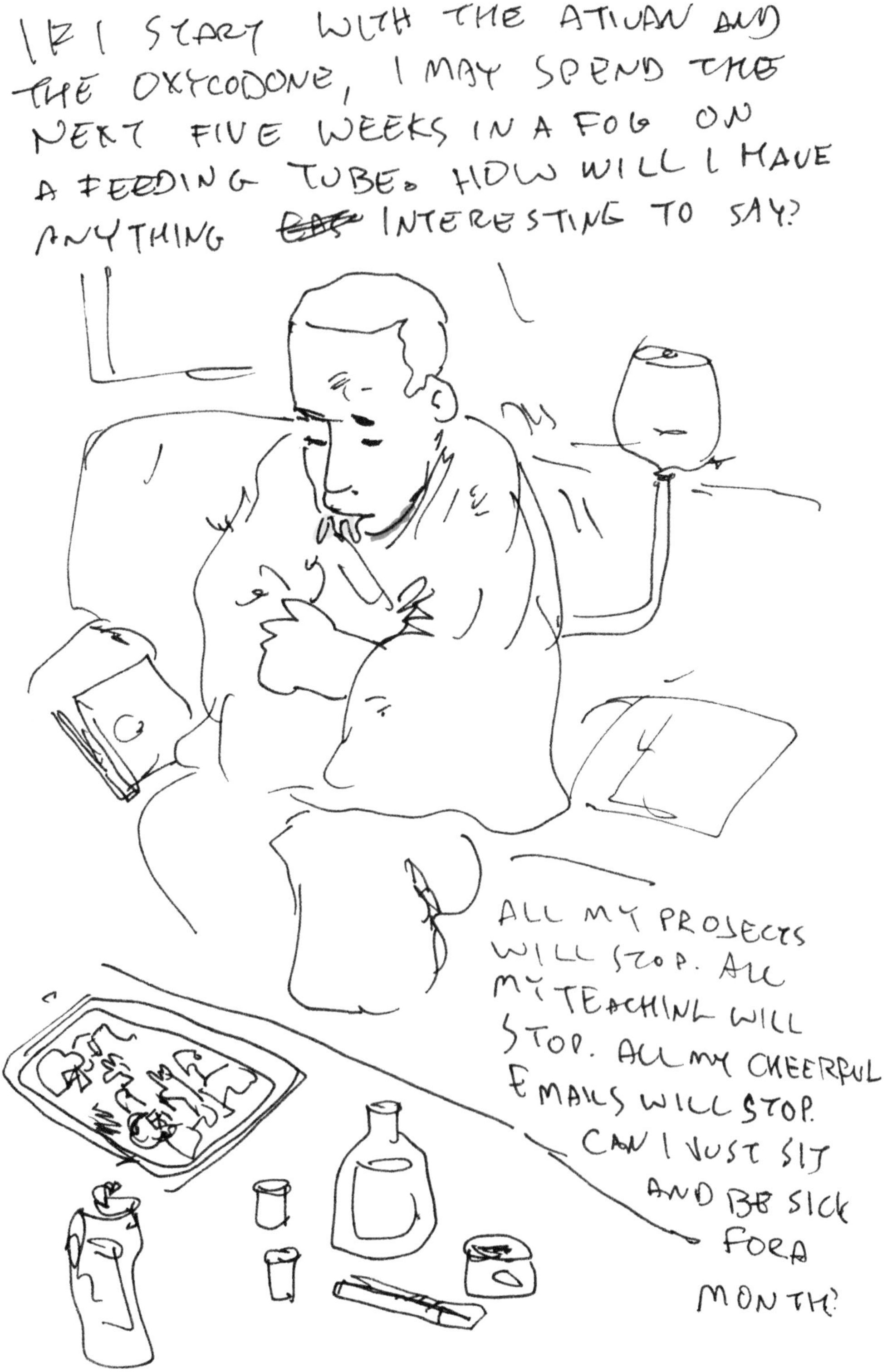
IF I START WITH THE ATIVAN AND THE OXYCODONE, I MAY SPEND THE NEXT FIVE WEEKS IN A FOG ON A FEEDING TUBE. HOW WILL I HAVE ANYTHING INTERESTING TO SAY?
ALL MY PROJECTS WILL STOP. ALL MY TEACHING WILL STOP. ALL MY CHEERFUL EMAILS WILL STOP. CAN I JUST SIT AND BE SICK FOR A MONTH?

DAY 11

YESTERDAY OTIS REDDING
VERY POPULAR
TODAY WILL BE JAMES
BROWN, "HELL"

YESTERDAY PARKING
SLOT 320. PET RUNNELS
WON THE AL BATTING
TITLE IN 1960 BATTING 320.
I HAD HIS CARD WITH THE HOUSTON
COLT .45's. HE WAS KIND OF
A LOST BATTING CHAMP IN BOSTON,
STUCK BETWEEN TED AND YAZ.
I IDENTIFIED WITH HIM AS A KID.

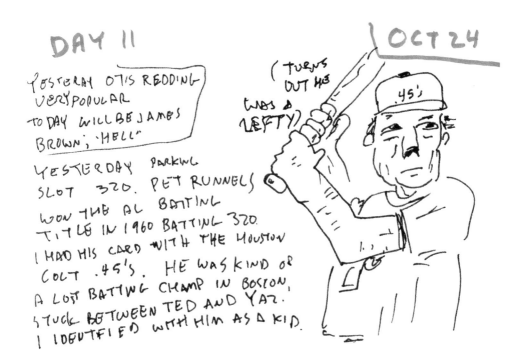

(TURNS OUT HE WAS A LEFTY)

WAITING FOR WEIGH-IN. FIRST SINCE
EATING BECAME AN ORDEAL. WAITING TO
SEE IF I'M LOSING WEIGHT. LAST NIGHT
I HAD MY FIRST INVALID MEAL, PICKING
UP TINY PIECES OF FISH AND BAKED
POTATOES AND YAMS AND FORCING THEM DOWN
TOPPED OFF WITH A CASHEW ALMOND SHAKE.
I WENT TO BED LAST
NIGHT PRETTY DISCOURAGED
ABOUT WHAT WAS
SHAPING UP FOR THE
NEXT FIVE WEEKS.

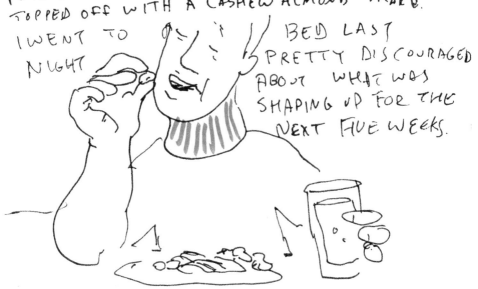

BUT THIS MORNING I FELT BETTER.
AS MY FRIEND TIM SAID THIS EVENING,
EVERYTHING THAT HAPPENED WAS PRE-
DICTED. THAT I WOULD FEEL BETTER
FOR A FEW DAYS THEN I WOULD CRASH
AS THE STEROIDS WORE OFF AND THE
EFFECTS OF THE CHEMO BECAME APPARENT.
THE PHLEGM BUILT UP AND RADIATION
BECAME DIFFICULT. ALL THAT I SAID,
BUT FORGOT AS IT ACTUALLY HAPPENED
THERE IS NO SUBSTITUTE FOR EXPERIENCE

SO TODAY TURNED OUT TO BE A
GOOD DAY. I WAS TOLD THEY
WOULD HAPPEN TOO, BUT I FORGOT.

IT'S HELL!

JAMES BROWN
WAS NOT VERY
CALMING, BUT I
WAS ABLE TO
FOCUS.

I CLOSED MY EYES AS SOON AS THE MASK
WENT ON. THAT HELPED. I TRIED TO FOCUS
ON EVERY BREATH. I HAD NO LIQUID IN MY
THROAT FOR THE FIRST 2/3 OF THE SESSION
BUT AS SOON AS THE FIRST DROP APPEARED
MY WHOLE BODY SPASMED AS ADRENALINE
SHOT FROM HEAD TO TOE. I HAD TO STRUGGLE
TO REGAIN CONTROL OF MY BREATHING AND
CALM BACK DOWN. I GUESS THAT'S WHY
THEY KEEP SUGGESTING ATIVAN. FOR
THE REST OF THE SESSION I WORKED HARD
TO KEEP CONTROL AND NOT LET MY
MIND WANDER. THAT KIND OF FOCUS IS UNNAT-

URAL FOR ME. I TAKE IT ALMOST AS
A POINT OF PRIDE THAT I CANNOT TRAIN
MY ATTENTION ON ANY SINGLE IDEA OR
OBJECTIVE FOR MORE THAN A FEW MOMENTS
AT A TIME. TO LOSE MYSELF IN THE WORK
I DO IS TO LOSE MY IDENTITY. THIS IS
OF COURSE THE EXACT OPPOSITE OF
WHAT YOU WANT TO HAPPEN DURING THE
CREATIVE PROCESS AND NATURALLY THE
OPPOSITE OF WHAT I TRY TO HELP MY STUDENTS
ACHIEVE.

THE LONGER I PLAYED BASEBALL, THE
MORE I THOUGHT AND THE WORSE I GOT.

STRIKE
THREE!

2-2 FIRST PITCH FASTBALL
      SECOND PITCH CURVE
0 0   THEN A FASTBALL
      THEN A CURVE
      SO IT SHOULD BE A
      FASTBALL OR MAYBE
      HE EXPECTS ME TO
      EXPECT A FASTBALL
      SO HE'S GOING TO THROW
      A CURVE. OR MAYBE
      HE EXPECTS ME TO EXPECT
      HIM TO CROSS ME UP.

WHEN I TRIED TO
WRITE I COULD ONLY
FOCUS FOR 45 MINUTES
AT A TIME. WHICH
MEANT IT WAS HARD
TO DEVELOP LONG
STORY ARCS.

RADIO
PLAYING

DISTRACTING
BOOKS, MAGAZINES
INTERNET
ALWAYS
AVAILABLE

100 STORIES
IN 100 DAYS

3 DAY NOVEL

FOOD ALL THE TIME

ONE NOVEL ABOUT
A 24 HOUR DAY

BATH-
ROOM
BREAKS
EVERY
20 MINUTES

4 PAGE A DAY GRAPHIC
PROJECT ABOUT CANCER
EXPERIENCE

MOM FLEW IN THIS AFTERNOON AND
JOINED US FOR MY SECOND CHEMO
SESSION. SO DID MY OLD COLLEGE
ROOMMATE JACK.

WE SAT FOR THREE HOURS. THE ROOM
HAD THE SAME VIEW AS THE HEALING GARDEN.

I GOT LOADED UP WITH A MOUTH OF
FREEZING MOUTHWASH TODAY AND A
SYRUP OF OXYCODONE AND ACETAMINOPHEN
SO I'M WELL ARMED FOR THE TROUBLES
AHEAD. I'M PREPARED NOW TO BECOME
A ZOMBIE IF NEED BE FOR THE NEXT
MONTH OR SO.

BITE OF COD, SPOON OF
SOUR CREAM, LADLE OF BROCCOLI, SPOON OF
SOUR CREAM. I'LL HAVE A FATAL HEART
ATTACK BEFORE I DIE OF CANCER.

DAY 12 WHEN THIS SESSION IS DONE I WILL BE JUST PAST THE $\frac{1}{3}$ MARK ON MY 35 DAY SCHEDULE.

OCT 25

TOM WAITS ON CD

STALL 52 FOR CAR

WILLIE MAYS HR TOTAL IN 1965

EASY ONE SHOT DAY UNFORTUNATELY JOVIAL TECH PHIL TRAUMATIZED MOM BY TRYING TO GOAD HER INTO MANUVERING THE GANTRY INTO POSITION WHEN ALL SHE WANTED TO DO WAS HOLD MY HAND.

THIS I NOT- BESIDES ROD, UNDER MY CHIN SEEMED TO BE GETTING LOOSE, TOO

MORNING ICED THAT GETTING THE SKIN

THIS IS ANOTHER THING PREDICTED
FOR THIS PROCEDURE: TURKEY WATTLE
NECK

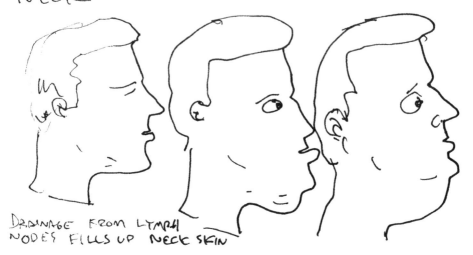

DRAINAGE FROM LYMPH
NODES FILLS UP NECK SKIN

MORE THINGS FOR MY MIND TO
WORRY VAINLY ABOUT.

SURVIVING CANCER IS ONE THING. SURVIVING
IT WITHOUT LOOKING LIKE A GHOUL IS
ANOTHER. BESIDES TURKEY NECK I COULD
END UP WITH

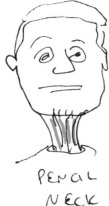

PENAL
NECK

MUSCLE ATROPHIES
AND DOESN'T COME
BACK

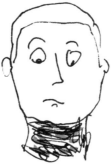

DISCOLORED
NECK
RADIATION
SUNBURN
PERMANENTLY
STAINS NECK

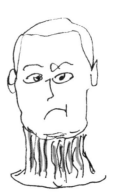

DROOPY
NECK

LOOSE SKIN
NEVER TIGHTENS
BACK UP

THIS AFTERNOON I SPENT AN HOUR WAITING FOR A CT SCAN OF MY CHEST TO CHECK ON THE PROGRESS OF THE NEGLECTED TUMORS IN MY LUNGS. I SAT NEXT TO A NICE WOMAN WHO WAS ALSO WAITING FOR HER SCAN.

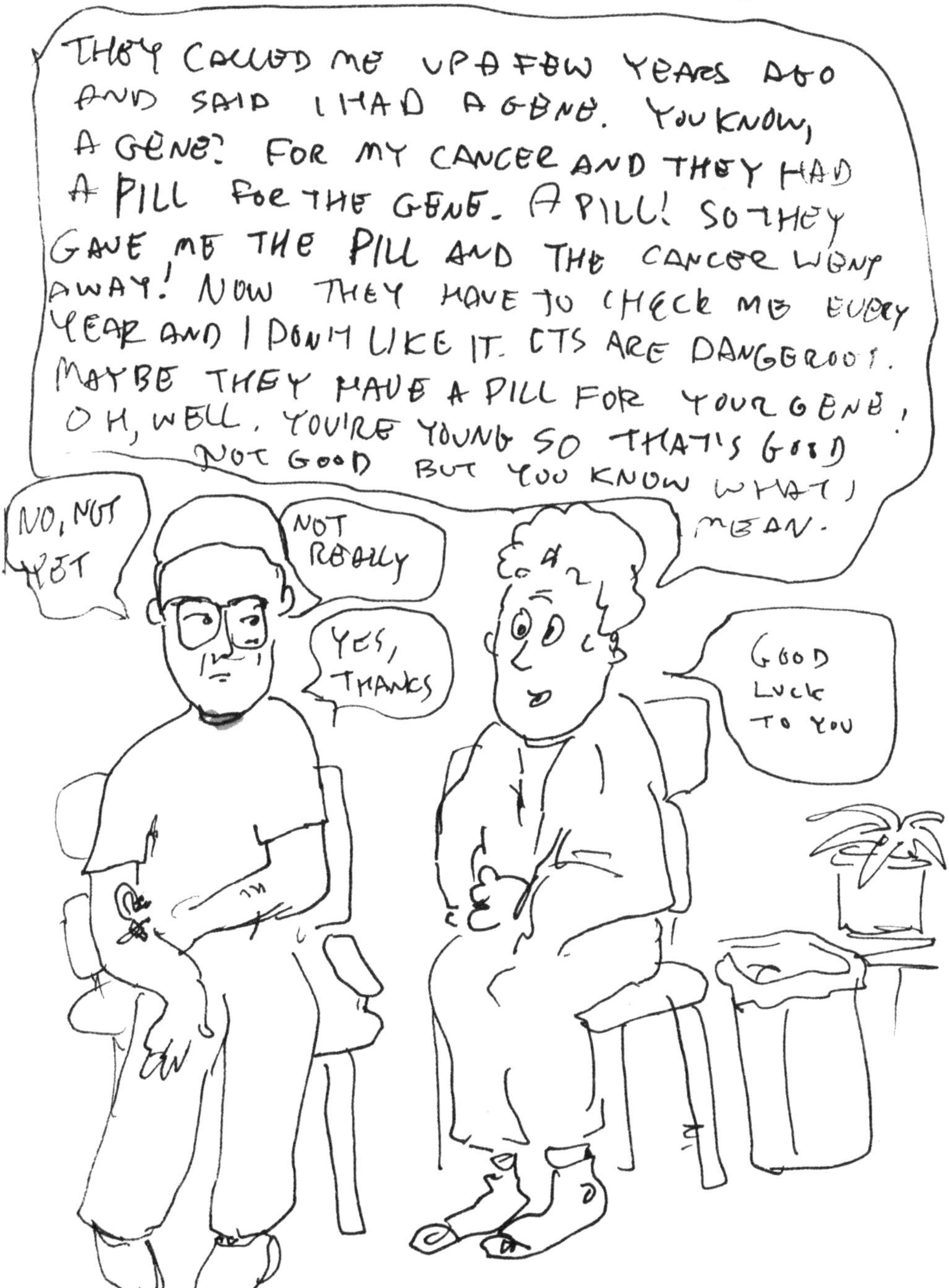

DAY 13

LAST NIGHT I WAS WORKING LATE TO COMPLETE MY FOUR PAGES AND I SKIPPED THESE TWO PAGES. SINCE I'M ON THE ALERT FOR SIGNS OF DETERIORATION, THIS IS NOT A GOOD SIGN.

4 MORE WAKE-UPS LAST NIGHT WITH DRY MOUTH AND THE NEED TO PEE. I FELT WOBBLY AND NAUSEATED FOR THE FIRST TIME THIS MORNING. I'M STAYING ON THE ZOFRAN.

I'M GETTING BETTER ABOUT FOCUSING MY BRAIN ON OTHER THINGS DURING RADIATION AND I GOT THROUGH IT OKAY. STILL, KATHY THE NURSE THINKS I AM COVERING UP TOO MUCH PAIN. I THINK SHE WANTS ME TO GO ON A PATCH THAT WILL MAINTAIN A STEADY LEVEL OF NARCOTIC PAIN RELIEF.

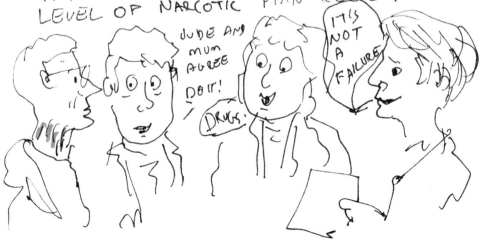

SO THIS EVENING I PUT A PATCH ON.
NOW I'M ALMOST ALL THE WAY INTO
ZOMBIE HOOD.

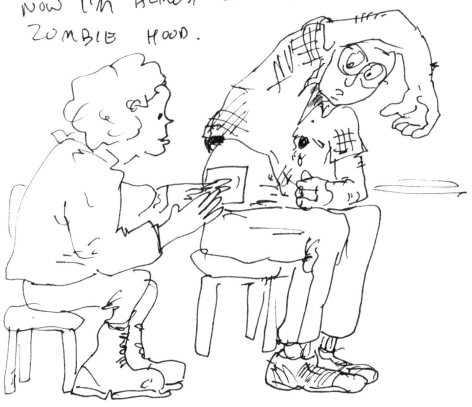

FIRST : NO DRUGS.
THEN : ACETAMINOPHEN
THEN : ROXICET, ACETAMINOPHEN + OXYCODONE
THEN : THE PATCH
NEXT : ATIVAN?

I WAS HOPING TO BE A CAREFUL OBSERVER
OF MY TREATMENT SO I WANTED AS CLEAR
A HEAD AS POSSIBLE TO REPORT ON WHAT
WAS HAPPENING TO ME. NOW AS THE SYMPTOMS
PILE UP I AM BECOMING AN ARTIFACT OF
MY OWN TREATMENT NEEDS AND MY ENTRIES
WILL REFLECT MY DETERIORATING ALERTNESS,
NOT SO MUCH MY PHYSICAL EXPERIENCE.

THIS EVENING WE WENT TO SEE OHINO! PHOTOS BY MY OLD FRIEND SOONI FROM COLLEGE WHO IS SHOWING HER NEW MOVIE AND PHOTOGRAPHS OF HER PARSIS COMMUNITY AT HARVARD.

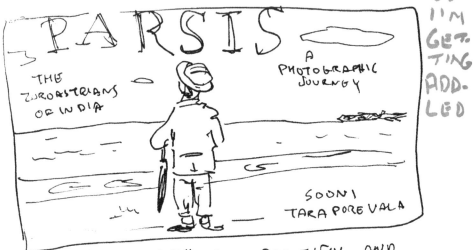

PARSIS

THE ZOROASTRIANS OF INDIA

A PHOTOGRAPHIC JOURNEY

SOONI TARA PORE VALA

THE PHOTOGRAPHS ARE BEAUTIFUL AND IT WAS GREAT TO SEE SOONI AGAIN.

AFTERWARDS THERE WAS A NICE RECEPTION WITH AN OPEN BAR AND LOTS OF DELICIOUS FOOD. PEOPLE DRINKING BEER AND WINE AND EATING CRACKERS AND CARROTS! THAT WAS THE MOST EXOTIC THING I SAW ALL EVENING.

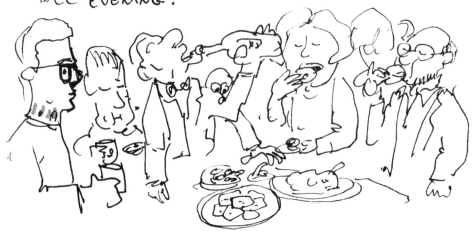

PARKED AT
STALL 270 TODAY.
NO ONE HAS HIT
EXACTLY 270
HOME RUNS.
PLAYED MY
FRIEND JEANNE'S
PIANO CD DURING
RADIATION. IT WAS
NICE TO HAVE A
FRIEND IN THE ROOM.

I ASKED JUDE FOR
A MANTRA THIS MORNING.
SHE TOLD ME SOMETHING
LONG IN SANSKRIT AND
I ASKED FOR SOMETHING
SHORTER AND SHE SAID
"GANA PATYUM YA" OR
SOMETHING LIKE THAT.
BUT I COULDN'T REMEMBER
IT TOO WELL. SO
I TRIED TO EXPERIMENT.

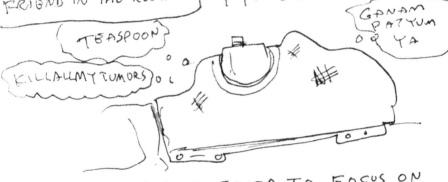

TEASPOON

KILL ALL MY TUMORS

GANAM PATYUM OR YA

FINALLY, I JUST TRIED TO FOCUS ON
BREATHING THROUGH MY NOSE.

THIS FRIDAY EVENING MY GROWING FEAR
IS THAT I AM BECOMING NAUSEATED. IF
I THROW UP I'M AFRAID THE GAME IS
UP AND IT WILL SOON BE THE TUBE
FOR ME. SPIT IS FILLING MY MOUTH,
I FEEL LIKE THROWING UP. MY TONGUE
IS FRIED BACON. I CAN'T POOP. MY HEAD
IS FULL OF COTTON. AND I'M WORRIED
ABOUT THE ELECTION TOO.

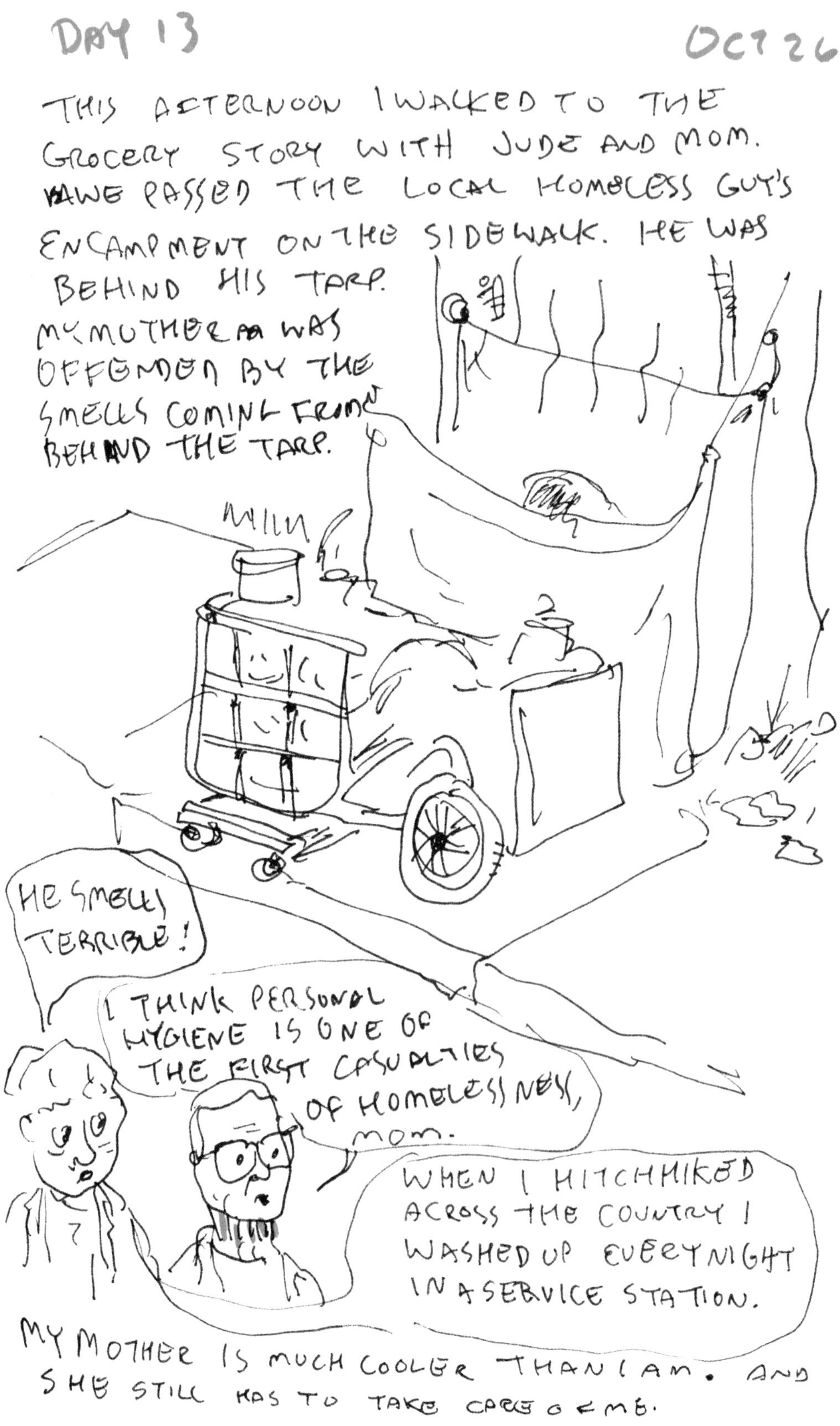
DAY 13
OCT 26
THIS AFTERNOON I WALKED TO THE GROCERY STORY WITH JUDE AND MOM. WE PASSED THE LOCAL HOMELESS GUY'S ENCAMPMENT ON THE SIDEWALK. HE WAS BEHIND HIS TARP.
MY MOTHER WAS OFFENDED BY THE SMELLS COMING FROM BEHIND THE TARP.
HE SMELLS TERRIBLE!
I THINK PERSONAL HYGIENE IS ONE OF THE FIRST CASUALTIES OF HOMELESSNESS, MOM.
WHEN I HITCHHIKED ACROSS THE COUNTRY I WASHED UP EVERY NIGHT IN A SERVICE STATION.
MY MOTHER IS MUCH COOLER THAN I AM. AND SHE STILL HAS TO TAKE CARE OF ME.

IN THE NEW YORK PAPERS THE NEWS
IS PREOCCUPIED WITH AN AWFUL STORY
ABOUT A NANNY WHO APPARENTLY KILLED
TWO CHILDREN AND THEN SLIT HER OWN
THROAT. THE CHILDREN'S MOTHER DISCOVERED
THEM. THEY WERE IN THE BATHTUB

LAST NIGHT I HAD A DREAM THAT
SOMEHOW I HAD MURDERED A FAMILY WHILE
OUT OF MY MIND ON ALL THESE PAIN
MEDICATIONS AND MY FAMILY AND JUDE
STILL HAD TO DECIDE IF THEY WOULD
TAKE CARE OF ME. THEY DID TAKE
CARE OF ME.
IN MANY WAYS BEING SICK IS EASY.
THE SICKER I FEEL, THE LESS I HAVE
TO DO. JUDE AND MOM FEED ME, DRIVE
ME, CLEAN UP AFTER ME, ENCOURAGE ME,
TELL ME TO TAKE IT EASY. ALL I HAVE TO
DO IS EAT

GOOD MATT!
EAT EVERYTHING!
HAVE ANOTHER BITE
MORE CARROTS
GOOD BOY!

THIS MORNING I HAD NO VOICE. THIS
IS A NEW ONE. I ONLY HAD TO GET UP
TWICE DURING THE NIGHT, WHICH WAS NICE,
BUT THE UNEXPECTED BAD NEWS TO THAT
GOOD NEWS WAS THAT MY THROAT AND TONGUE
WERE DRIER THAN EVER. THIS MORNING
MY TONGUE LOOKS LIKE A TATOOED
STAR WARS VILLIAN

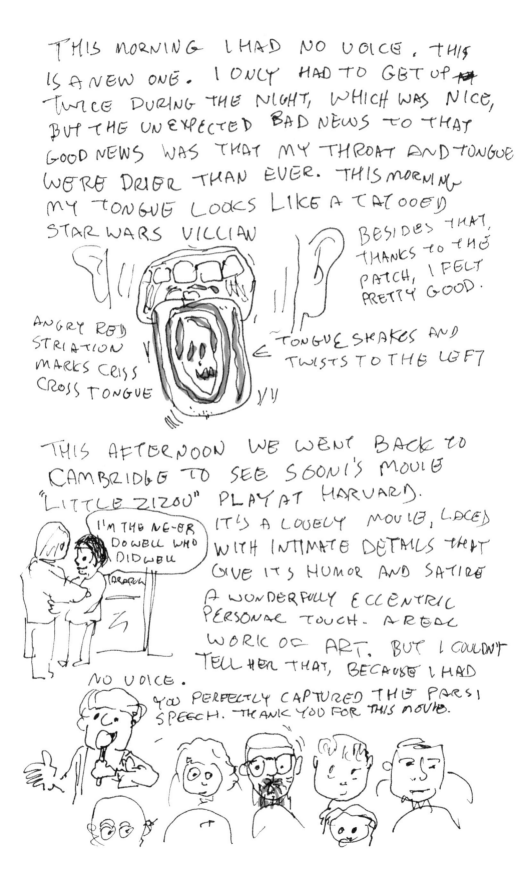

BESIDES THAT,
THANKS TO THE
PATCH, I FELT
PRETTY GOOD.

ANGRY RED
STRIATION
MARKS CRISS
CROSS TONGUE

TONGUE SHAKES AND
TWISTS TO THE LEFT

THIS AFTERNOON WE WENT BACK TO
CAMBRIDGE TO SEE SOONI'S MOVIE
"LITTLE ZIZOU" PLAY AT HARVARD.
IT'S A LOVELY MOVIE, LACED
WITH INTIMATE DETAILS THAT
GIVE ITS HUMOR AND SATIRE
A WONDERFULLY ECCENTRIC
PERSONAL TOUCH. A REAL
WORK OF ART. BUT I COULDN'T
TELL HER THAT, BECAUSE I HAD
NO VOICE.

I'M THE NE-ER
DO WELL WHO
DID WELL

TARAPORE

YOU PERFECTLY CAPTURED THE PARSI
SPEECH. THANK YOU FOR THIS MOVIE.

JUDE IS LEAVING TOMORROW AND
MOM IS ALREADY MOVING TO CONSOLIDATE
HER DIETARY ADVANTAGE. WHEN WE WENT
TO THE STORE SHE BOUGHT CHICKEN,
CHICKEN STOCK AND STEAK TO MAKE SOME
KIND OF KILLER CHICKEN SOUP OUT OF.
JUDE IS BEING VERY COOL ABOUT THINGS.

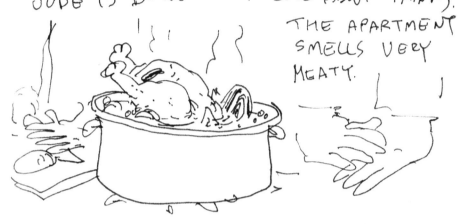

THE APARTMENT
SMELLS VERY
MEATY.

THERE IS ALSO A DIFFERENCE OF OPINION
OVER ENSURE VS. NUT SHAKES.

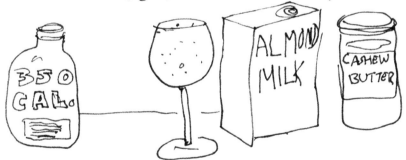

JUDE IS VERY SUSPICIOUS OF THE SUGARS
AND OBSCURE CHEMICALS THAT GIVE
ENSURE ALL ITS PUNCH AND CONVENIENCE.
MOM TRUSTS THE MEDICAL ESTABLISHMENT
AND ENSURE IS ON THE APPROVED LIST OF
FOODS THEY GAVE ME WHEN I GOT HERE.
I'LL EAT OR DRINK ANYTHING I CAN
SWALLOW. I WISH I HAD STRONGER
FEELINGS ON THE ISSUE, BUT I JUST DON'T.

OCT 28 | I DID IT AGAIN, MISSED TWO
PAGES LAST NIGHT WHILE TRYING
TO FILL UP MY PAGES. I THINK I STILL HAVE
MY MARBLES BUT THEY'RE SLIPPING AWAY.
TOOK ME TWO MINUTES THIS MORNING
TO REMEMBER ALL MY NIECES + NEPHEW'S NAMES.

JUDE IS PACKING TO GO BACK THIS MORNING
FLEURRY IS GOING TOO.
LAST NIGHT AT 2 AM MOM WAS
COOKING MORE CHICKEN SOUP AND CLEANING
THE KITCHEN FLOOR WITH A PAPER TOWEL.

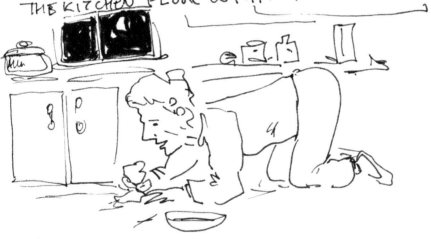

NOW I JUST HAD TO LOOK UP "TRANSFORMERS!"

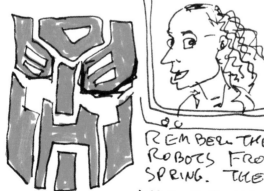

A TV COMMENTATOR
MENTIONED
"AUTOBOTS"
AND "DECEPTICONS"
AND I COULDN'T
REMEMBER THE MIGHTY RACE OF
ROBOTS FROM WHENCE THEY
SPRING. THE CLOSEST I CAME
WAS "CONVERTIBLE ROBOTS".

OCT 28 | THIS MORNING WE DROVE OUT TO BOXFORD MASSACHUSETTS TO PICK UP A CAR MY OLD COLLEGE ROOMMATE JACK IS LENDING US FOR THE REST OF MY TREATMENT. FOR 23 YEARS JACK HAS BEEN BUILDING, PLANTING, LANDSCAPING, PAINTING, CARVING AND MASSAGING THE PLACE AND ITS SURROUNDING ACRES TO FIT HIS VISION. I'VE NEVER BEEN HERE BEFORE. THAT'S MY FAULT.

JACK + MICHIKO'S HOUSE

IRONWOOD TREE

STONE + BRICK PATH LAID BY JACK.

JAPANESE PEAR TREE

MICHIKO, JACK'S WIFE

DAWN REDWOOD PLANTED BY JACK

SWAMP RECLAIMED BY JACK.

SLIDING

← REGLAZED BY JACK

DOOR + WINDOW LINE UP

JACK

JACK

BARN BUILT BY JACK FROM TREES GROWN BY JACK. PLANED AND PINNED BY JACK. WALLS RAISED BY JACK AND HIS NEIGHBORS.

WE HAD TO GO TO THE HARVARD
COOP TO BUY A NEW BOOKBAG FOR
ME — OVERSTUFFING WITH MY SHELF FULL OF
MEDICINES FINALLY GOT TO IT. WE WENT
BY MY OLD FRESHMAN DORM, WIGGLESWORTH.
WHAT A NAME. I FELT NOTHING. NOT A TINGLE.

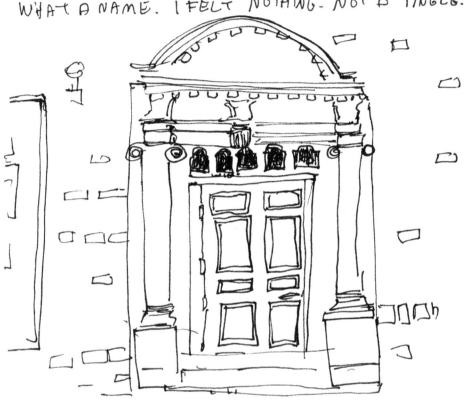

BUT THEN AFTER I BOUGHT THE BOOKBAG
I WANDERED INTO THE COOPS' CLOTHING SECTION.
I SAW A HARVARD CREW HAT. I PICKED IT UP, THEN
PUT IT DOWN AND, LEFT THE SECTION. THEN I
CAME BACK AND ~~CAME~~ PICKED UP THE HAT
AND BOUGHT IT. SO, I'M NOT SO COOL

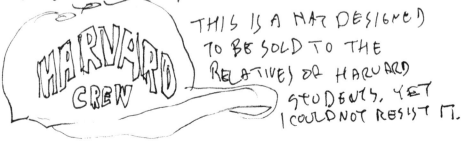

THIS IS A HAT DESIGNED
TO BE SOLD TO THE
RELATIVES OF HARVARD
STUDENTS, YET
I COULD NOT RESIST IT.

THE BIG STORM IS COMING
SO JUDE DROVE BACK TO NYC
AND I DROVE BACK TO BOSTON WITH MOM.
I HAD TO USE THE GPS IN MY PHONE TO
NAVIGATE HOME. MOM AND I AREN'T NECESSARILY
COMPATIBLE DRIVING COMPANIONS.

THAT CAR DIDN'T USE ITS TURN SIGNAL

NOT WHAT I'D CALL A CONSIDERATE DRIVER —

— YES AND I REALLY DON'T LIKE PEOPLE WHO USE THOSE DEVICES WHILE DRIVING. JUST THROW IT AWAY AND KEEP YOUR HANDS AT NINE AND THREE O'CLOCK.

MOM, I CAN DRIVE!

I KNOW I SHOULD USE BOTH HANDS BUT I KIND OF AM BEING A JERK.

WE GOT HOME OKAY. BUT JUDE, DRIVING
BACK WITH FLEURRY GOT CAUGHT IN
SLOW TRAFFIC. FERRIES AND TUNNELS
AND BRIDGES ARE BEING CLOSED UP AND
DOWN THE EAST COAST. WE CHARGED
OUR BATTERIES, FILLED BUCKETS WITH WATER,
COLLECTED MATCHES AND CANDLES, AND
WAITED TO HEAR IF
JUDE AND FLEURRY MADE IT
HOME. I COULD IMAGINE
JUDE GETTING STUCK ON
THE WRONG SIDE OF THE WHITESTONE
BRIDGE, LIVING FOR DAYS IN AN EVACUEE CAMP
IN ~~TENNESSEE~~ CONNECTICUT, RIDING OUT THE WORST
STORM IN A CENTURY. AT LEAST
SHE HAS
FLEURRY.

(I WROTE TENNESSEE THERE. WHY?)

SUPPOSE I CAN'T GO INTO
THERAPY IN THE MORNING? SUPPOSE I CAN'T
GO ALL WEEK? DO ALL THE TUMORS GROW BACK?
RADIATION THERAPY IS SUPPOSED TO BE A
ROUTINE. A WHOLE DIFFERENT KIND OF CRISIS
LAID ON TOP OF A REGULAR CRISIS.
I'M TOO DRUGGED UP TO FULLY APPRECIATE
WHAT THIS STORM COULD DO, BUT I KNOW
THE SYNAGOGUE COULD FLOOD IF THE

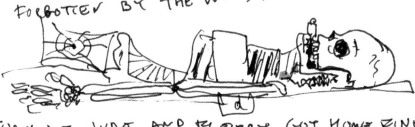

TOILETS BACK UP AND THE DRAINS FAIL. WE
COULD LOSE ALL OUR WORK.
THE HOUSE IN CHILMARK COULD BLOW AWAY

WE COULD LOSE ALL OUR MONEY.

PEWER COULD FAIL IN THE HOSPITAL AND
THE STAFF COULD FLEE LEAVING ME STRAPPED
TO THE TABLE IN THE PROTON ROOM FOR MONTHS,
FORGOTTEN BY THE WORLD.

TURNS OUT, JUDE AND FLEURY GOT HOME FINE.

STILL 297

RICKEY HENDERSON   JOHN COLTRAN CD
HIT 297 HOMERS

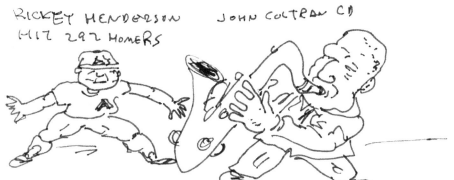

IN THE MIDDLE OF THE NIGHT I HAD SOME
KIND OF WEIRD DREAM THAT SEEMED TO CONFLATE
THE ELECTORAL COLLEGE WITH ARITHMATIC
ABOUT FRACTIONS OF THERAPY LEFT. I DRIFTED
IN AND OUT OF CONSCIOUSNESS, TRING TO FIGURE OUT
HOW MANY DAYS WERE LEFT IN THERAPY AND HOW
TO GET TO 270 ELECTORAL VOTES.

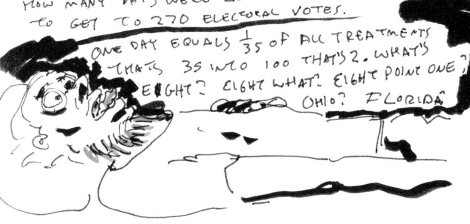

ONE DAY EQUALS $\frac{1}{35}$ OF ALL TREATMENTS
THATS 35 INTO 100 THAT'S 2. WHAT'S
EIGHT? EIGHT WHAT? EIGHT POINT ONE?
OHIO? FLORIDA?

AT SOME POINT BARACK OBAMA HIMSELF
BECAME INVOLVED I THINK...

ACTUALLY, I THINK HE
WAS NUMBER CRUNCHING.
THESE
ARE
WEIRD
DRUGS.

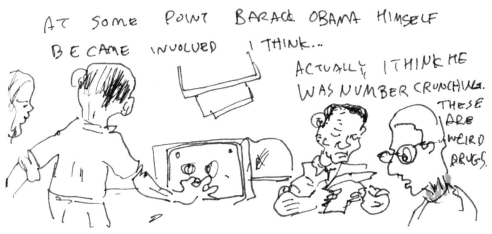

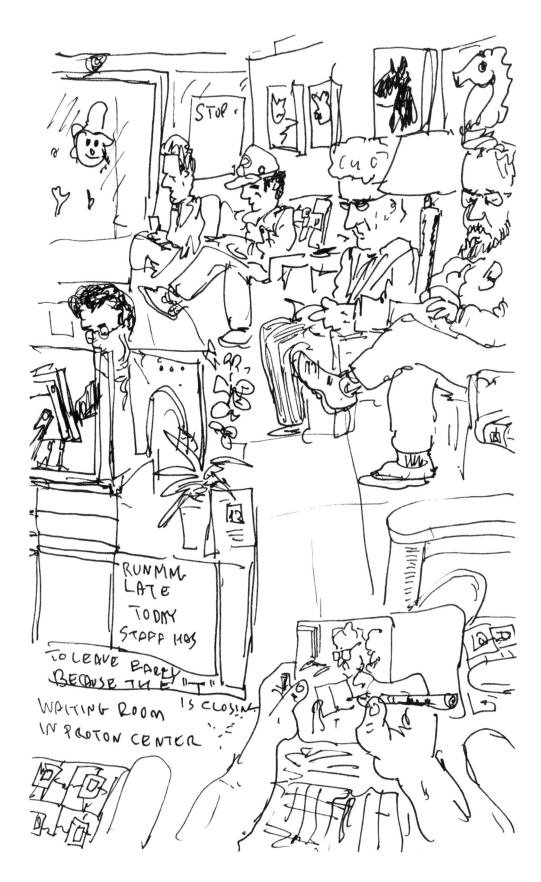

WE GOT HOME OKAY IN THE RAIN AND
WENT IMMEDIATELY TO WHOLE FOODS, THE
CLOSEST STORE. WE BOUGHT A GALLON OF WATER
AND SOME PUMPKIN IN A CAN, BUT THE MAJORITY
OF OUR PURCHASES WERE PREOCCUPIED WITH MY
EATING LIMITATIONS AND WERE HIGHLY DEPENDENT ON
ELECTRIC TECHNOLOGY.

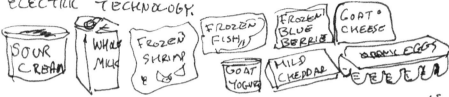

ABOUT $250 OF GROCERIES, MOSTLY PERISHABLE.

THEN TO WALGREENS FOR SHAMPOO
ENERGY DRINKS, PRUNES AND TRICK
OR TREAT CANDY. WE WEREN'T
EXACTLY PREPARING FOR THE STORM
OF THE CENTURY.

MY MOUTH WAS REALLY BURNED BY
THE TREATMENT TODAY AND EATING A
BOWL OF SOUP WAS ABOUT THE HARDEST
THING I HAVE EVER DONE. ONE TINY
SPOONFUL OF SOUP, A SWIG OF MAGIC
MOUTHWASH, ANOTHER SPOONFULL OF SOUP,
SOME OXYCODONE ACETAMINOPHEN SYRUP,
AND SO ON. IN THE MEAN TIME,
THE RADIO BROADCAST, THE REAL
NEWS OF THE DAY.

"SUBWAYS AND TUNNELS CLOSED IN NEW YORK."

"EVACUATION OF LOW LYING AREAS."

THOUSAND MILE STORM FROM" NINE STATES
DECLARE STATE OF EMERGENCY. OBAMA AND
ROMNEY SUSPEND CAMPAIGN ACTIVITIES"
BUT I WAS FOCUSED ON MY SOUP.

THEN OF COURSE, RIGHT ABOUT FOUR PM.

THE POWER GOES OUT.

SO MOM AND I PUT OUR COATS BACK ON AND TRUDGED BACK TO THE WALGREENS. THIS TIME TO BUY BATTERIES OR MAYBE A RADIO THAT DIDN'T NEED TO BE PLUGGED IN. NATURALLY. IT WAS CLOSED THEY TOLD US THEY WOULD SHUT DOWN AS SOON AS THE POWER FAILED.

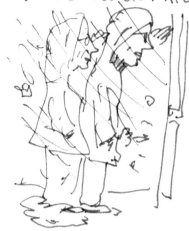

OUR INVENTORY OF AVAILABLE COMMUNICATION DEVICES IS TWO MOSTLY CHARGED PHONES. A MOSTLY CHARGED IPAD AND A MOSTLY CHARGED LAP TOP.

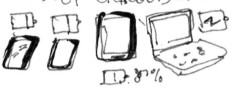

THAT SHOULD BE ENOUGH FOR A WHILE, RIGHT? BUT I'M DOLING OUT USE LIKE IT'S WATER IN A LIFEBOAT.

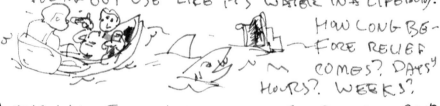

HOW LONG BEFORE RELIEF COMES? DAYS? HOURS? WEEKS?

LUCKILY ELLEN IS VERY SPIRITUAL AND THERE ARE LOTS OF CANDLES. OR MAYBE SHE IS JUST VERY EMERGENCY SAVVY.

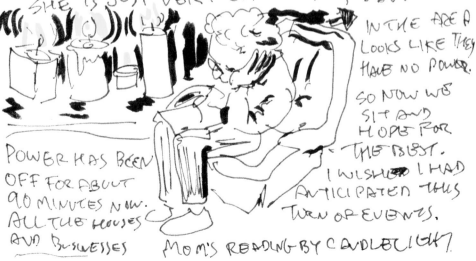

IN THE AREA LOOKS LIKE THEY HAVE NO POWER.

SO NOW WE SIT AND HOPE FOR THE BEST. I WISHED I HAD ANTICIPATED THIS TURN OF EVENTS.

POWER HAS BEEN OFF FOR ABOUT 90 MINUTES NOW. ALL THE HOUSES AND BUSINESSES

MOM'S READING BY CANDLELIGHT.

THE POWER WENT OUT AND HAS STAYED OUT. WE ARE MEMBERS OF THE 300,000 CUSTOMER TRIBE WITHOUT POWER IN MASSACHUSETTS.

THE 'GOUE IN NYC IS FINE. JUST A FEW SHINGLES OFF THE ROOF. THE EXTENSIVE HURRICANE PREPAREDNESS WAS UNNECCOSSARY.

MASS   MY WAS FINE

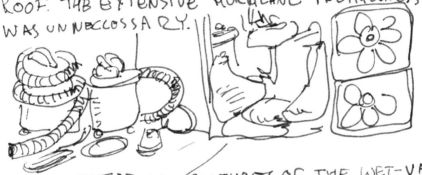

JUDE TEXTED ME PICTURES OF THE WET-VACS, EXTENSION CORDS AND SUMP PUMPS ALL PRIMED AND READY TO GO. ALSO THE SANDBAGS IN THE DOORWAYS TO THE BATHROOMS AND THE FANS STACKED AND PREPARED TO BLOW AWAY THE FLOOD. THEN NOTHING.

WHILE WE SAT IN NEWTON AND WAITED FOR THE FROZEN SHRIMP TO MELT. MY BIG CHALLENGE WAS TO EAT A BOWL OF CHICKEN SOUP BY CANDLELIGHT. IT TOOK ABOUT AN HOUR TO GET IT ALL DOWN. BUT I DID! MEANWHILE, IN NYC THE VIEW FROM BILL'S WINDOW ON 12TH ST.

THIS MORNING JUDY RESCUED US AGAIN. SHE HAULED ALL THE COLD FOOD OVER TO HER HOUSE AND DROVE US TO THE HOSPITAL.

MOM SEEMED ODDLY RELUCTANT TO LEAVE THE POWERLESS HOUSE AND MORE WILLING TO TAKE CHANCES WITH THE FOOD THAN I WOULD HAVE THOUGHT.

THIS EGG IS STILL COOL. DOESN'T IT FEEL COOL?

IT FEELS PRETTY COOL

A CHILLED GEL?

I'M NOT WORRIED IN ENGLAND THEY USED TO EAT EGGS THAT SAT IN SOME KIND OF CHILLED GEL.

EVERYTHING WAS WORSE IN ENGLAND AFTER THE WAR. WE WERE THERE FOR ABOUT A YEAR.

I FORGET MOM COMES FROM PIONEER STOCK, ONE OF THE FEW JEWISH HOMESTEADERS IN KANSAS

HER GRANDMOTHER GAVE BIRTH TO CHILDREN ALL BY HERSELF IN THEIR SOD HOUSE.

HER GRAND FATHER USED TO WALK 30 MILES FOR WORK IN FT DODGE.

WAH! WAH! IN FT DODGE.

ONCE SHE CHASED OFF AN EAGLE THAT TRIED TO STEAL MY GREAT UNCLE HENRY.

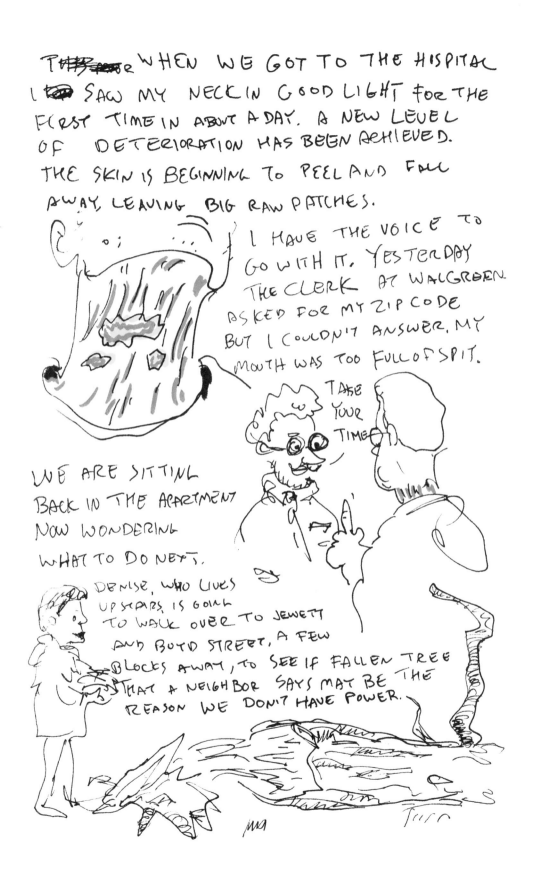

~~THERE~~ WHEN WE GOT TO THE HOSPITAL
~~I SAW~~ SAW MY NECK IN GOOD LIGHT FOR THE
FIRST TIME IN ABOUT A DAY. A NEW LEVEL
OF DETERIORATION HAS BEEN ACHIEVED.
THE SKIN IS BEGINNING TO PEEL AND FALL
AWAY, LEAVING BIG RAW PATCHES.

I HAVE THE VOICE TO
GO WITH IT. YESTERDAY
THE CLERK AT WALGREEN
ASKED FOR MY ZIP CODE
BUT I COULDN'T ANSWER. MY
MOUTH WAS TOO FULL OF SPIT.

TAKE YOUR TIME

WE ARE SITTING
BACK IN THE APARTMENT
NOW WONDERING

WHAT TO DO NEXT.

DENISE, WHO LIVES
UPSTAIRS, IS GOING
TO WALK OVER TO JEWETT
AND BOYD STREET, A FEW
BLOCKS AWAY, TO SEE IF FALLEN TREE
THAT A NEIGHBOR SAYS MAY BE THE
REASON WE DON'T HAVE POWER.

MOM IS IN THE KITCHEN NOW COOKING SOME TALAPIA WE FORGOT TO BRING OVER TO JUDY'S THIS MORNING. AND I AM GOING TO EAT IT.

CAN YOU SMELL ANYTHING?

NO---

MOM ATE THE FISH FIRST, THEN I ATE SOME. SO FAR SO GOOD. SHE ALSO MADE STEWED APPLES AND STEWED PRUNES. I'M TRYING TO PACK ON WEIGHT FOR TOMORROW'S SESSION WITH DRS. BENDAPUDI AND WIRTH. IF I'VE LOST TOO MUCH WEIGHT IT'S THE TUBE FOR ME.

AT 4:29 PM WHILE WE WERE TALKING TO MY BROTHER BART, THE POWER CAME BACK ON WITH A POP.

WHEN WILL THE POWER COME BACK?

DAY 16

IT'S HALLOWEEN. I PLAN ON WEARING MY COMIC FLASHING LED TEETH TO MEETINGS WITH DOCTORS AND RADIATION THERAPY TODAY. WE'LL SEE HOW THAT GOES OVER. MEANWHILE I'M WAITING TO GET WEIGHED. I'M WEARING MY HEAVIEST CLOTHES.

FLANNEL LINED JEANS

HEAVY WOOL HIKING SOCKS

EXTRA SHIRT

OF COURSE THE REAL QUESTION IS WHETHER TRYING TO GAME THE SYSTEM HELPS ME OR HURTS ME.

THE TONGUE BATTLE MAP. HAS EVOLVED INTO A EUROPEAN

I'M CONCERNED THAT MY TONGUE POSITION UNDER THE BITE BLOCK HAS EXPOSED IT TO TOO MUCH RADIATION

MOTTLED PURPLE INTERIORS (DULL ACHE)

BITE BLOCK

TONGUE

TO MUCH

BRIGHT RED LINES (SHARP PAIN)

TIP LOOKS NORMAL, BUT TINGLES

I THINK THE TONGUE IS SUPPOSED TO LIE FLAT UNDER THE BITE BLOCK. AS TIME HAS GONE ON AND MY JAW HAS GOTTEN TIGHTER, MY TONGUE HAS GOTTEN SORER AND MY BEHAVIOR DURING RADIATION HAS GOTTEN MORE DELIBERATE. I HAVE BEEN MANUEVERING THE BITE BLOCK WITH MY TONGUE TO ALLOW ME TO BREATHE WITHOUT GAGGING.

TONGUE

BITE BLOCK

TUMOR

I SLIGHTLY CURL AND TENSE THE TONGUE TO CREATE A SMALL AIR PASSAGE BELOW THE BITE BLOCK. THIS BRINGS MY TONGUE BACK AND UP A BIT. DOES THIS PUT THE TIP IN LINE FOR TOO MUCH RADIATION? OR DOES EVERYTHING GO TO THE BACK WHERE THE TUMOR IS?

WEIGHT STABLE AT 184 SO ANOTHER WEEK WITHOUT THE TUBE WARNED AGAIN THAT IT IS STILL OUT THERE WAITING FOR ME SO NO GLOATING ALLOWED. THEY WANT ME TO BE EVEN MORE DOPED UP THAN I AM. I'M SUSPECTED OF BEING TOO MACHO AND PRIDEFUL THAN IS GOOD FOR ME.

NO MED RADIATION THERAPY = TRIP TO HEAVEN

PATCHES NARCOTICS IV FEEDING

TUBE = TRIP TO HELL

I AM WORRIED ABOUT THE DRUGS, IF ONLY BECAUSE I HATE BEING IN A FOG. THE INCENTIVE OF THE DRS. UNDERSTANDABLY IS SIMPLY TO GET ME THROUGH THE THERAPY. MY ENJOYMENT OF THE THERAPY, OR MORE ACCURATELY MY EXPERIENCE OF THE THERAPY OR MORE ACCURATELY MY CONSCIOUSNESS DURING THE THERAPY IS SECONDARY. I THINK THEY WOULD BE HAPPY TO CYROGENICALLY FREEZE THEIR PATIENTS FOR TWO MONTHS AND WAKE THEM UP WHEN IT'S ALL OVER.

BUT NOW WHAT THE HELL. I'LL SPEND THE NEXT FOUR WEEKS IN A STUPOR.

OCT XXXX   NOV XXXX

BACK ON CHEMO DRIP NOW I HAVE BECOME COMFORTABLY NUMB.

MOM WALKED OVER TO THE HEALING GARDEN
AT THE END OF THE HALL AND BROUGHT BACK

IT'S A HEALING STONE

PICK ONE HAND

SO NOW I HAVE THAT
GOING FOR ME.
A NICE LADY WITH A THICK
BOSTON ACCENT IS BEHIND
THE NEXT CURTAIN
TALKING TO ALL HER FAMILY
AND FRIENDS.

ALL THESE
PEOPLE I DON'T
EVEN KNOW
KEEP PRAYIN'
TO GAWD I'LL
BE OKAY.

YORE MY
SISTAH.
NUFF SAID
WE STAHT
OVAH AGAIN
NOW.

THIS
AFTER-
NOON I ATE
A SMALL CUP OF
VANILLA ICE CREAM
IT WAS THE MOST DISTURBING 4 OZ. OF FOOD
I'VE EVER CONSUMED IN MY LIFE. THE MATERIAL
I CONSUMED HAD THREE AND ONLY THREE QUALITIES
1. EXTREME COLD, COLD ALMOST INDISTINGUISHABLE FROM
   EXTREME HEAT.
2. SAND-LIKE GRAININESS
3. THE DENSITY OF THICK MUD

I FORCED MYSELF THROUGH JUST
TO GET THE CALORIES, BUT IT
MADE ME REALIZE THAT TASTE IS HIGHLY
DEPENDENT ON EXPECTATION. IF IT HAD BEEN
LABLED "FROZEN SAND MUD" I PROBABLY
WOULDN'T HAVE TOUCHED IT, CALORIES
OR NO, BUT I FORCED MYSELF TO FINISH IT
BECAUSE, ICE CREAM, I DEEPLY BELIEVE,
IS GOOD. NOW THAT THAT LAST ILLUSION
HAS BEEN TAKEN FROM ME, I WILL NEVER TRUST

VANILLA
ICE CREA

LUV PLEASUM

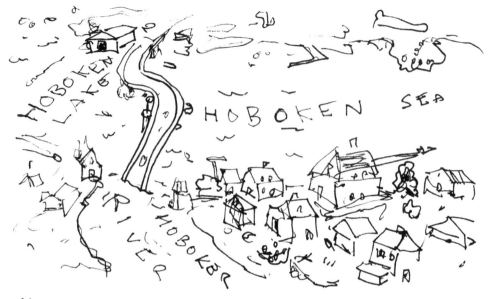

HOBOKEN LAKE

HOBOKEN SEA

HOBOKEN

HOBOKEN RIVER

MEANWHILE MY FRIENDS IN NEW JERSEY ARE UNDER WATER. I'M GOING TO BE HERE FOR A MONTH. WHEN I GET BACK TO NEW YORK WILL THE SUBWAYS BE RUNNING, POWER BACK ON EVERYWHERE, STREETS CLEANED, CELL PHONES FUNCTIONING? IT TURNS THE BAD DREAM OF THIS CANCER TREATMENT UPSIDE DOWN.

I'M SORT OF CLOSING MY EYES AND HOPING THE CANCER WILL BE GONE WHEN I OPEN THEM. NOW I'M ALSO HOPING THAT NEW YORK, ETC. WILL BE THE SAME. ONLY NOT- AS THEY WERE BEFORE. MAYBE THE CRYOGENIC FREEZE ISN'T SUCH A BAD IDEA.

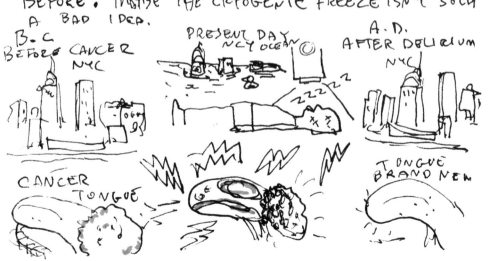

B.C
BEFORE CANCER
NYC

PRESENT DAY
NYC OCEAN

A.D.
AFTER DELIRIUM
NYC

CANCER
TONGUE

TONGUE
BRAND NEW

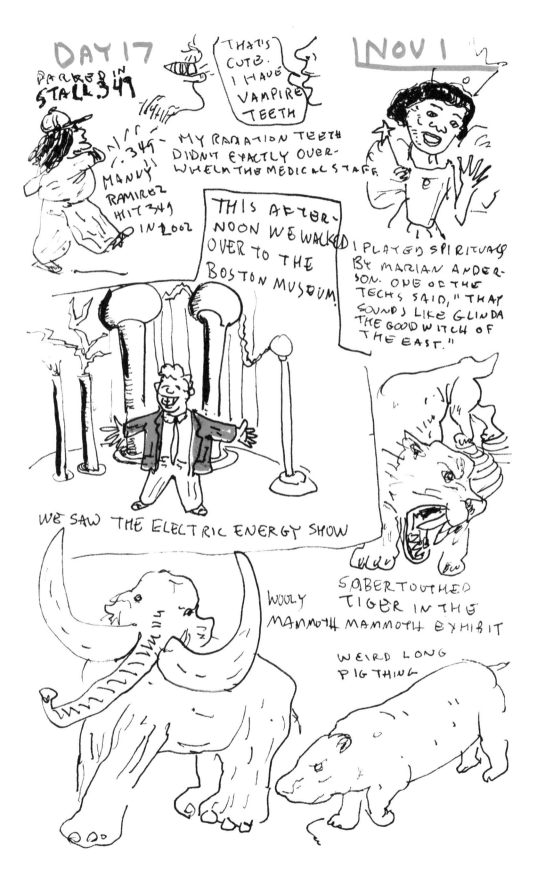

AFTERWARD WE WENT INTO THE
BUTTERFLY ROOM. IT WAS VERY PEACEFUL.

OWL
BUTTER-
FLY

DEAD
BUTTERFLY
ON FLOOR

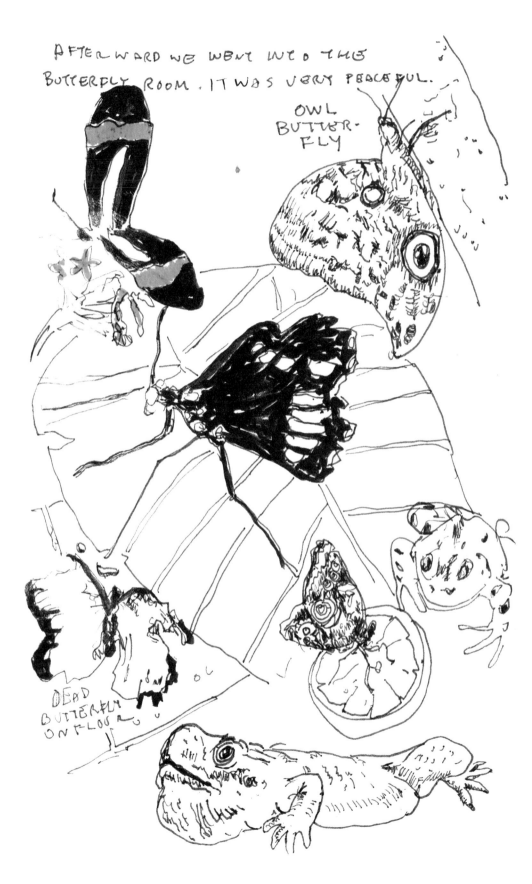

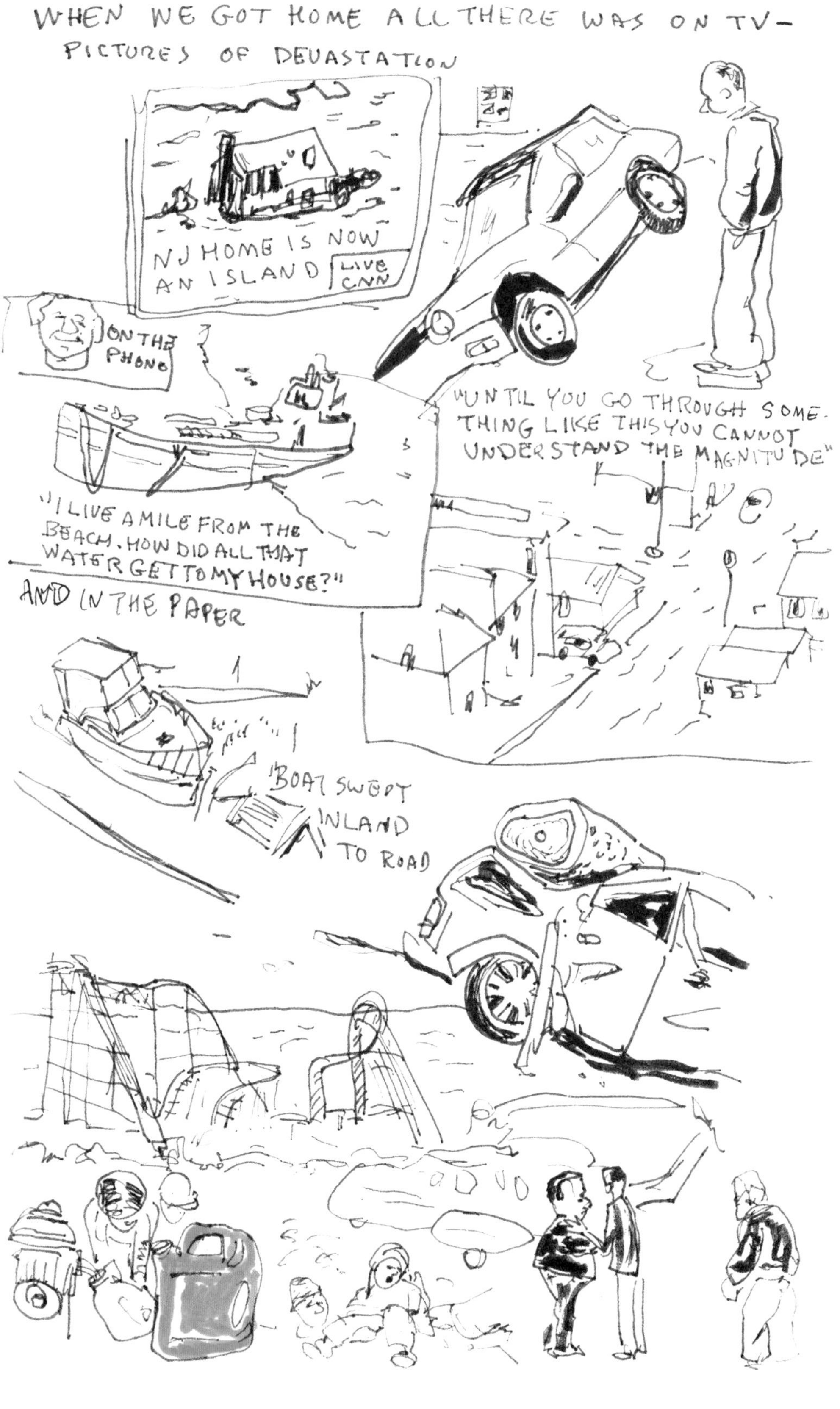

WHEN WE GOT HOME ALL THERE WAS ON TV—
PICTURES OF DEVASTATION

NJ HOME IS NOW
AN ISLAND

LIVE CNN

ON THE
PHONE

"UNTIL YOU GO THROUGH SOME-
THING LIKE THIS YOU CANNOT
UNDERSTAND THE MAGNITUDE"

"I LIVE A MILE FROM THE
BEACH. HOW DID ALL THAT
WATER GET TO MY HOUSE?"

AND IN THE PAPER

"BOAT SWEPT
INLAND
TO ROAD"

BUT THEN I HAD DINNER AND EVERYTHING SHRUNK DOWN TO NOTHING AGAIN. I'M NEARLY HALF WAY DONE. BUT IT FELT LIKE THIS EVENING I REALLY DID FALL OFF A CLIFF.

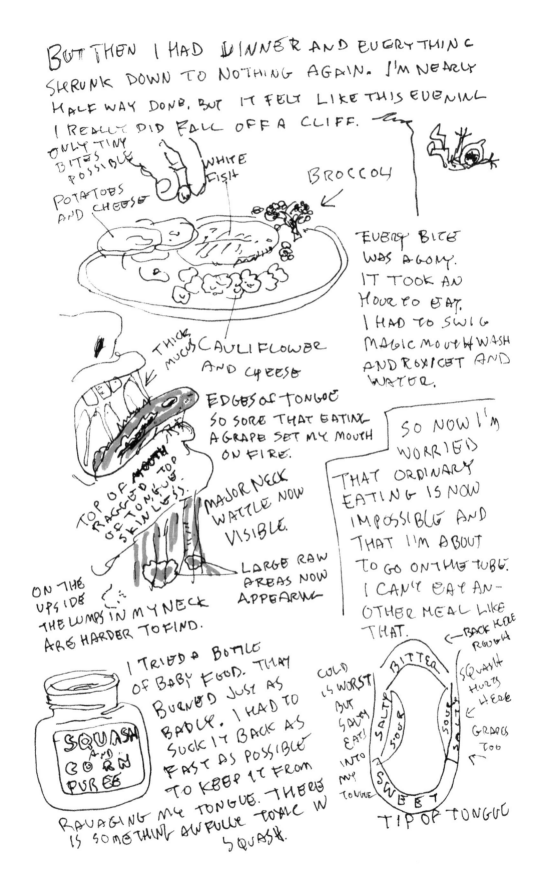

ONLY TINY BITES POSSIBLE

WHITE FISH

POTATOES AND CHEESE

BROCCOLI

EVERY BITE WAS AGONY. IT TOOK AN HOUR TO EAT. I HAD TO SWIG MAGIC MOUTHWASH AND ROXICET AND WATER.

THICK, MUCUS CAULIFLOWER AND CHEESE

EDGES OF TONGUE SO SORE THAT EATING A GRAPE SET MY MOUTH ON FIRE.

TOP OF MOUTH RAGGED. TOP OF TONGUE SKINLESS.

MAJOR NECK WATTLE NOW VISIBLE.

LARGE RAW AREAS NOW APPEARING

ON THE UPSIDE THE LUMPS IN MY NECK ARE HARDER TO FIND.

SO NOW I'M WORRIED THAT ORDINARY EATING IS NOW IMPOSSIBLE AND THAT I'M ABOUT TO GO ON THE TUBE. I CAN'T EAT AN- OTHER MEAL LIKE THAT.

I TRIED A BOTTLE OF BABY FOOD. THAT BURNED JUST AS BADLY. I HAD TO SUCK IT BACK AS FAST AS POSSIBLE TO KEEP IT FROM RAVAGING MY TONGUE. THERE IS SOMETHING AWFULLY TOXIC IN SQUASH.

SQUASH AND CORN PUREE

COLD IS WORST BUT SOUR EATS INTO MY TONGUE

BITTER

SALTY SOUR

SWEET

BACK HERE ROUGH

SQUASH HURTS HERE

GRAPES TOO

TIP OF TONGUE

DAY 18 WHEN I AM IN THE MIDDLE OF TODAY'S THERAPY I WILL [NOV 2]

BE EXACTLY ½ OF THE WAY THROUGH TREATMENT. I AM TOO SUPERSTICIOUS TO ADD AN EXCLAIMATION POINT TO THE END OF THAT LAST SENTENCE. THE QUESTION, AGAIN, IS WHAT KIND OF PLACE AM I AT— THE TOP OF THE MOUNTAIN AND IT'S ALL DOWN — HILL FROM HERE OR THAT GODDAMNED CLIFF OFF OF WHICH I KEEP THINKING I HAVE JUST FALLEN. LAST NIGHT WITH THE **HORRIBLE DINNER** I WAS CONVINCED IT WAS THE CLIFF, TODAY WITH SOME SLEEP AND MEDS, THINGS ARE SLIGHTLY LOOKING UP. WHATEVER ELSE THIS MEANS, I THINK MY HEAD IS NOW FIRMLY UP MY ASS FOR THE DURATION, AND NOTHING, NOT WORLD CHANGING FLOODS, CIVIC BREAK DOWN, A PRESIDENTIAL ELECTION, COMPLETE LOSS OF CONTACT WITH MY WIFE, MY FAMILY, MY STUDENTS, MY JOB—IS GOING TO WREST MY ATTENTION FROM MY ROSTER OF COMPLAINTS : SORE NECK, INEDIBLE FOOD, FEAR OF FEEDING TUBE.

THE REAL WORLD BELONGS TO THE "HEALTHIES" AND IT'S THEIR PROBLEM. I GET A FREE PASS TO WORRY ABOUT NOTHING BUT MYSELF. IT HARDLY SEEMS FAIR. I THINK I WILL SEND MONEY TO THE [+] TO ASSUAGE MY GUILT. PAUL DROVE OFF TODAY TOWARDS WOODSTOCK. HE CAN'T GET INTO JERSEY CITY, WHERE HE WORKS, BECAUSE THE ROADS ARE FLOODED. HE CAN'T GO SEE HIS SON IN MANHATTAN BECAUSE OF THE BAN ON CARS WITH LESS THAN THREE PASSENGERS. HE DOESN'T KNOW IF HIS HOUSE IN WOODSTOCK STILL EXISTS.

STRANGE TIMES. THE WORLD IS SHRINKING TO THIS LITTLE BOOK 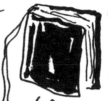 AND THE FOUR PAGES A DAY I'M ASSIGNED BY MYSELF TO FILL. I WORRY ABOUT THOSE PAGES BUT I ALSO LOOK FORWARD TO THEM. THEY ARE THE ONLY CONCRETE, SATISFYING THING I DO NOW. I HAVEN'T LOOKED BACK MUCH TO WHAT I WROTE EARLIER. AND I DOUBT I WILL EVER READ THE WHOLE BOOK AT ALL ONCE IT IS FINISHED UNLESS I AM FORCED TO BY CIRCUMSTANCE, BUT I KNOW IT HAS TIGHTENED UP FORMWISE AND GOTTEN MORE STUFFED WITH DATA AS THE WORLD AROUND ME OR AT LEAST MY ENGAGEMENT IN THE WORLD SHRINKS. IT IS STARTING TO TAKE OVER MY LIFE, OR RATHER MY LIFE IS STARTING TO SHRINK TO THE SIZE OF THIS NOTEBOOK. I DON'T KNOW WHAT I'D DO IF I LOST IT. THIS FOLLOWS THE STANDARD SEQUENCE FOR A PROJECT AT LEAST FOR ME. (DID I ALREADY WRITE ABOUT THIS? CAN'T REMEMBER. DRUGS?)

PROJECT FOCUS ↑

5 DAYS   10 DAYS   15 DAYS   TODAY   FUTURE?

TIME →

EVERY SUSTAINED ART PROJECT GRINDS SLOWLY, THEN HITS SOME KIND OF RHYTHM → THE ELUSIVE "FLOW" THAT CREATES THE ILLUSION OF MAGICAL, EFFORTLESS WORK AND CREATES ITS OWN SELF SUSTAINING REASON FOR CONTINUING TO WORK: THE ADDICTIVE PHASE. THEN AS YOU GRIND ON, BEGIN TO TIRE, BEGIN TO AWAKEN FROM YOUR DAZE OF PRODUCTIVITY. THINGS FLOW OUT MORE SLOWLY AND IN LESS COMPELLING WAYS UNTIL YOU ARE FINALLY JUST REPEATING OLD TRICKS. THEN YOU STOP. THE BELL CURVE OF ART IN THIS CASE THERE IS   BAD GOOD BAD   THERE IS ALSO THE DANGER OF

THE BRAGG CURVE OF ART MIMICKING THE PROTON THERAPY. THERE IS ALSO, ALWAYS, THE DREAM OF

BAD ← MEDIOCRE

INTERESTING

① THE MAGIC SUSTAINED MANIA CURVE.

MAYBE THE "EUREKA" CURVE IN WHICH AN ARTIST ACHIEVES A BREAKTHROUGH IN THINKING OR EXPERIENCE OR COURAGE AND NEVER LOOKS BACK. I

INSIGHT? ACHIEVED

ONCE HEARD DAVID SMITH PUT EVERYTHING TOGETHER DURING A MONTH IN SPOLETO.

BUT WHO KNOWS?

I WONDER ABOUT THE GOD CURVE WHERE THINGS JUST GET BETTER AND BETTER AND MORE AWESOME FASTER AND FASTER FOREVER. I SUPPOSE

CURVE

GOODNESS

TIME

YOU ONLY WONDER ABOUT THE GOD CURVE WHEN YOU ARE ON DRUGS.

I SUPPOSE THERE IS ALSO THE LIFE : DEATH : ART CURVE. IN WHICH THE RACE AGAINST THE END IS AT ODDS WITH, SOMETIMES, THE ABILITY TO MAKE GOOD WORK. OR MAYBE JUST THE OPPOSITE.

?? MOZART 0.0001 % GRAPH ANALYSIS SHOWS HARDLY
EVERYBODY ELSE 96.9999% ANY LIKELIHOOD OF ME
BAD POETS 3% BEING FAVORABLY AFFECTED BY REALITY OR FEAR OF IMMINENT DEATH.

GOOD   BAD

LIKELIHOOD OF DEATH

SECOND PATCH ADDED THIS EVENING. NOW I'M TRULY WOOZY.

25 OK 12

YET DINNER WAS TORTURE 2.0 WAR CRIME.

BABY VANILLA YOGURT →

THE EXTRA 50% IN THE PATCH HAS KNOCKED ME OUT WITHOUT MAKING ME ANY MORE COMFORTABLE. A BAD COMBINATION. WOULD LIKE TO CELEBRATE HALFWAY POINT, BUT NOT FEELING TOO UPBEAT. ALL I CAN DO IS FOCUS ON THE NINE

3) TWEET

ROOF OF MOUTH —
BACK OF TONGUE
INSIDE OF GUMS (2)
SIDE OF TONGUE (2)
ROOT OF TONGUE
TOP OF TONGUE
BAND OF NECK SKIN

EXTRA! TIP OF TONGUE

POINTS OF PAIN IN MY HEAD RIGHT NOW. ACTUALLY, MAKE THAT TEN POINTS OF PAIN.

I WANT TO FOCUS ON SOMETHING OUTSIDE MY BODY, BUT I CANNOT.

I ONLY HAVE ROOM FOR THE PAINS IN MY HEAD. THIS AFTERNOON WE WALKED OVER TO THE LIBERTY HOTEL, WHICH IS ATTACHED TO THE HOSPITAL. IT'S A LUXURY HOTEL MADE OUT OF THE OLD CHARLES STREET JAIL. YOU CAN LOOK AT THE OLD CELLS ON YOUR WAY TO YOUR ROOM OR ONE OF THE MANY CAFES, WINE BARS OR RESTAURANTS ON THE PREMISES. TURNS OUT THE CUPOLA I KEEP TRYING TO DRAW WHEN I'M SITTING IN THE HEALING GARDEN IS THE TOP OF THE OLD JAIL/HOTEL.

JAIL

HEALING GARDEN
I WILL HAVE TO INVESTI-
GATE. IF I REMEMBER IN THE MORNING,

THIS WEEKEND OFF. CAME JUST IN TIME. NOV 3

THE HIGHER LEVEL OF DRUGS HAS NOT YET TRANSLATED INTO INTO LESS PAIN ON THE TONGUE AND IN THE MOUTH.

- LOTS OF DRUGS
- SOME DRUGS
- HARDLY ANY DRUGS

AND THIS MORNING THE OUTSIDE OF THE NECK REALLY BEGAN TO HURT. IT FEELS LIKE A RAZOR HAS BEEN DRAGGED ACROSS MY NECK.

THE SKIN AT THE CENTER OF THE NECK HAS DRIED UP AND IS BEGINNING TO SLOUGH OFF.

DEAD POTATO BUG NECK

CONFETTI NECK

MOST IMPRESSIVELY, THE PATTERN OF THE BURN HAS A VERY DISTINCT OUTLINE.

• MOSCOW

IT LOOKS LIKE THE MAP OF RUSSIA

A SMALL CONTROVERSY = HOW TO TREAT THE NECK

KEEP NECK DRY AND EXPOSED TO AIR.

COVER WITH AQUAPHOR AND BANDAGE.

THIS FEELS WORSE

THIS FEELS BETTER

DR. LIEBSCH

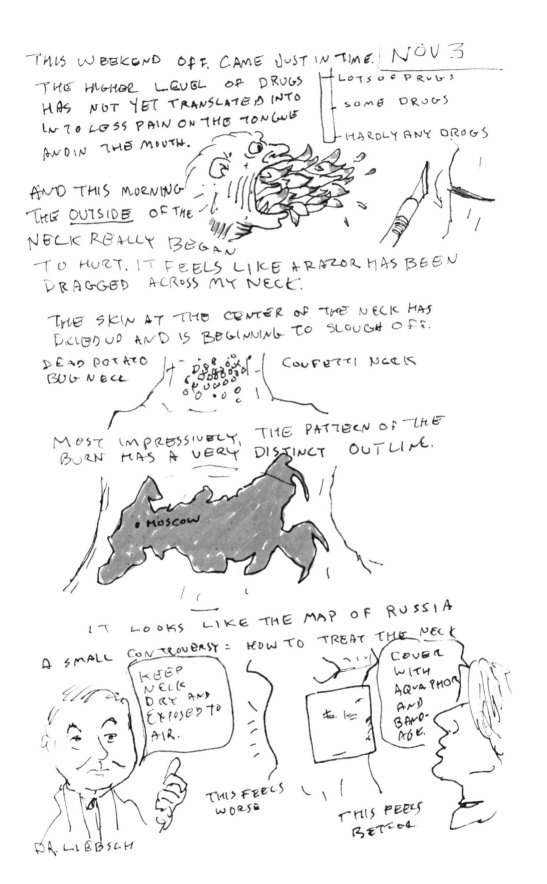

EVERYTHING I DO NOW IS FOCUSED ON DIVIDING AND PARSING THE PAIN IN MY MOUTH OR IN THE TIME LEFT IN SECONDS, MINUTES, HOURS, DAYS OR WEEKS, IN WHATEVER PARTICULAR ORDEAL I AM TRYING TO GET THROUGH.

INSIDE MY MASK DURING RADIATION I LISTEN FOR 1. THE WHIR OF THE PROTON BEAM MACHINE AS IT ROTATES INTO PLACE.

THEN 2. THE CLICKS AND SNAPS AS FIRST
A) THE BRASS DISC AND THEN
B) THE LUCITE DISC THAT

TOGETHER NARROW AND LIMIT THE BEAM ARE SNAPPED INTO PLACE.

A - T3

DON'T MOVE!

THEN 3.) THE NUMBERS AND LETTERS OF THIS PARTICULAR FIELD ARE CALLED OUT TO THE TECH IN THE NEXT ROOM.

4). THE TECH SAYS "HOLD STILL" AND THE DOOR CLOSES,

5) THEN THE HUM OF THE SPINNER THAT SPREADS THE BEAM BEGINS TO CRANK UP.

6) THE CLANKS OF THE MAGNETS THAT DIRECT THE BEAMS THROUGH THE TUBES FROM THE PROTON ACCELERATOR START TO CHATTER.

7) THE HUM GOES ON AND ON FOREVER SOMETIMES, AND MY MOUTH BEGINS TO TINGLE. I SWEAR I CAN FEEL IT. THEN FINALLY THE SPINNING SOUND SLOWS AND NOW WE ARE ALMOST OVER.

8) BEEP!

9) DOOR OPENS AND THE TECH WALKS BACK INTO THE ROOM.

AS ALL THIS IS GOING ON I'M TRYING TO KEEP MYSELF AS STILL AND CALM AS POSSIBLE. THE MESH HELMET MAKES IT POSSIBLE TO SEE A BIT OF WHAT IS GOING ON AROUND ME, AND AT FIRST I LIKED THE DISORIENTING FEELING OF WATCHING THE ROOM SPINNING AROUND ME. BUT AS TIME WENT ON AND THE MUCUS IN MY MOUTH GOT THICKER AND THICKER, ANY LOSS OF CONCENTRATION COULD START ME ON A CHOKING SPREE.

SO I CLOSE MY EYES AS SOON AS I LIE DOWN AND BEGIN TO BREATH THROUGH MY NOSE. I HAVE TO KEEP MY BREATH SHALLOW SO I DON'T GULP. IF I GULP, THEN FLUID BEGINS TO LEAK INO THE BACK OF MY NECK.

CALM

NO WATER - GOOD

ALERT

SOME WATER - OK

ALARM

SPASM

ENOUGH WATER TO GURGLE - BAD

I'M USUALLY OKAY FOR THE FIRST AND EVEN FOR THE SECOND "FIELD"- WHAT THEY CALL EACH RADIATION SEQUENCE- BUT BY THE THIRD THERE IS ALMOST ALWAYS A MOMENT WHEN I EITHER NOTICE THAT SOME WATER HAS BEGUN TO COLLECT IN MY NECK, OR I LOSE MY BREATHING FOCUS FOR A MOMENT AND I GASP AND GAG FOR AIR. THEN I HAVE TO BRING IT BACK UNDER CONTROL BY BREATHING SLOWER AND SLOWER AND FEELING FOR THE AIR PASSING BACK AND FORTH THROUGH MY NOSE. THAT CALMS ME DOWN AND HELPS ME FOCUS.

I'VE DONE YOGA EXERCISES FOR 15 YEARS AND MY BREATH CONTROL HAS ALWAYS BEEN TERRIBLE, BECAUSE I COULD GET AWAY WITH IT.

MY BREATH CONTROL NOW IS VERY ADVANCED BECAUSE IT HAS TO BE.

SNIFFER SNIFF SNIFF

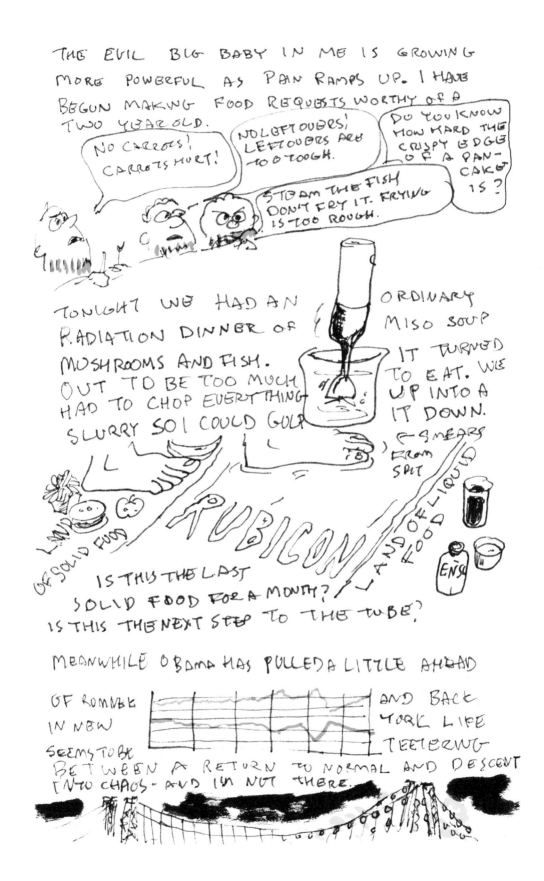

THE EVIL BIG BABY IN ME IS GROWING MORE POWERFUL AS PAIN RAMPS UP. I HAVE BEGUN MAKING FOOD REQUESTS WORTHY OF A TWO YEAR OLD.

NO CARROTS! CARROTS HURT!

NO LEFTOVERS! LEFTOVERS ARE TOO TOUGH.

DO YOU KNOW HOW HARD THE CRISPY EDGE OF A PAN-CAKE IS?

STEAM THE FISH DON'T FRY IT. FRYING IS TOO ROUGH.

TONIGHT WE HAD AN ORDINARY DINNER OF MISO SOUP MUSHROOMS AND FISH. IT TURNED OUT TO BE TOO MUCH TO EAT. WE HAD TO CHOP EVERYTHING UP INTO A SLURRY SO I COULD GULP IT DOWN.

R-SMEARS FROM SPIT

LAND OF SOLID FOOD   RUBICON   LAND OF LIQUID FOOD

ENSU

IS THIS THE LAST SOLID FOOD FOR A MONTH? IS THIS THE NEXT STEP TO THE TUBE?

MEANWHILE OBAMA HAS PULLED A LITTLE AHEAD OF ROMNEY AND BACK IN NEW YORK LIFE SEEMS TO BE TEETERING BETWEEN A RETURN TO NORMAL AND DESCENT INTO CHAOS - AND I'M NOT THERE.

SUNDAY MORNING. RAIN SOMEHOW RATCHETED UP OVER THE NIGHT. I WANT TO SEE THE WIDER WORLD BUT THE PAIN IN MY HEAD KEEPS ME HUNKERED DOWN AS IF I'M IN A WWI TRENCH.

THIS SUNDAY WAS A TERRIBLE DAY. THIS IS THE FIRST DAY THAT MAKES IT CLEAR I MAY NOT BE ABLE TO FORCE MY WAY THROUGH EVERYTHING. THE PAIN WON'T GO AWAY. EVEN MY OLD EAR PAIN HAS COME BACK. I'M GOING TO HAVE TO UP THE DOSAGE, BUT THE REALLY FRIGHTENING DISCOVERY IS THAT THE MAGIC MOUTHWASH IS NO LONGER MASKING THE PAIN IN MY TONGUE.

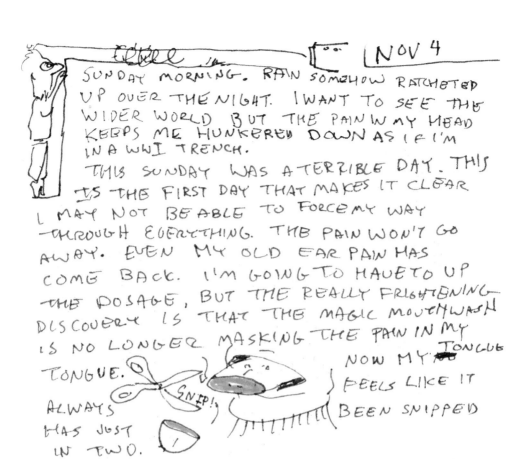

NOW MY TONGUE FEELS LIKE IT BEEN SNIPPED

ALWAYS HAS JUST IN TWO.

SNIP!

THIS CARTOON-Y FORMAT CREATES A BIAS TOWARDS HUMOR AND LIGHTHEARTEDNESS, BUT I DON'T FEEL LIKE THAT AT ALL.

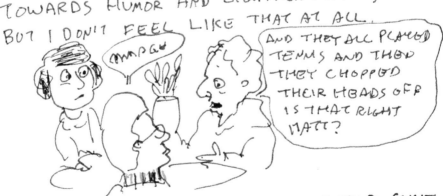

MMPGH

AND THEY ALL PLAYED TENNIS AND THEN THEY CHOPPED THEIR HEADS OFF IS THAT RIGHT MATT?

THIS AFTERNOON AN OLD FAMILY FRIEND CAME OVER TO VISIT AND I COULDN'T SPEAK. SO MY MOTHER HAD TO TELL HER WHAT ALL MY BROTHERS AND MY SISTER AND MY NIECES AND NEPHEWS WERE UP TO. EVERY TWO MINUTES I HAD TO LEAN OVER AND SPIT INTO A CUP.

TOMORROW MOM GOES BACK TO CHICAGO FOR A WEEK AND MY BROTHER BART ARRIVES FROM SEATTLE FOR A WEEK. BART IS A LOT MORE CASUAL THAN MOM. I'M SUCH A BABY NOW. I'M WORRIED HE WON'T KNOW HOW TO FEED ME PROPERLY.

MAYBE HE WILL FORCE ME TO EAT A STEAK.

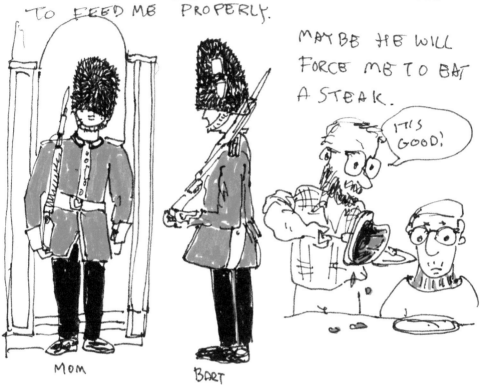

IT'S GOOD!

MOM

BART

THIS AFTERNOON WE WENT TO THE PHARMACY AND THE CLERK ASKED FOR MY ZIP CODE TO AUTHENTICATE MY CREDIT CARD. MY MOUTH WAS SO FILLED WITH SPIT THAT I COULDN'T TALK SO I HAD TO USE SIGN LANGUAGE. I FELT PRETTY SILLY. I THINK THIS IS THE NEW NORMAL, SO I BETTER GET USED TO IT.

EIGHT

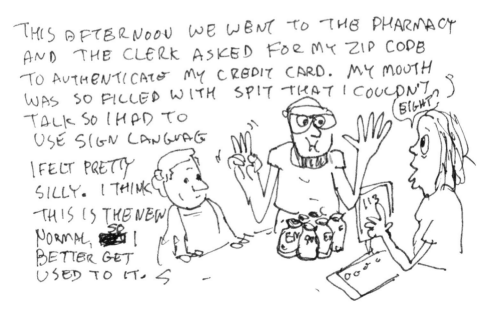

NOW I'VE LOST MY LAST GOOD PEN.
THE WHEELS BE FALLING OFF THE CART.

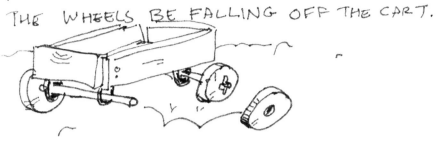

EVERYTHING LEADING UP TO THIS WAS
A JOKE. ALL THE BRAVADO WAS JUST
THAT. I KNEW IT, BUT I COULDN'T FEEL
IT. NOW I GOT IT ALL, THE PAIN, THE
FOGGINESS, THE ANGER, THE ENDLESS
STRETCH OF TIME BEFORE IT ENDS.
AND I HAVE NONE OF THE RESOURCES
LEFT TO COMBAT ALL THAT. EXCEPT
ONE THING: STUBBORNES. HOW LONG
WILL THAT LAST?

MY SISTER JOHANNA IS MAYBE EVEN
MORE STUBBORN THAN ME. ITS A MIR-
ACLE EITHER ONE OF US EVER DOES
ANYTHING, SINCE OUR STUBBORNESS IS
USUALLY IN DEFENSE OF INERTIA.

WHY'D THEY
SNIP THOSE
POLYPS? I
LOOKED THEM
UP AND THEY
WEREN'T
EVEN
PRE-CANCEROUS.

THEIR
SOLUTION
TO EVERY-
THING IS
"PUT ME
ON THE
TUBE!"
I DON'T
WANNA
BE ON
THE
TUBE.

I SPENT MOST OF THE DAY WATCHING
FOOTBALL GAMES ON TV.

THE BEARS WON AGAIN, BUT
I DOUBT THEY ARE ALL THAT
GOOD.

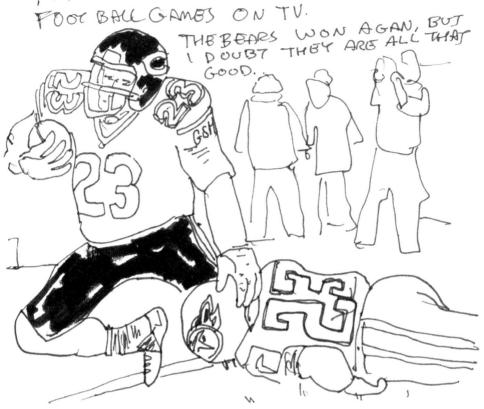

WE DID TAKE A WALK THIS AFTERNOON
TO SEE THE TREE THAT FELL DOWN AND
CAUSED THE BLACK OUT IN OUR NEIGHBOR-
HOOD.

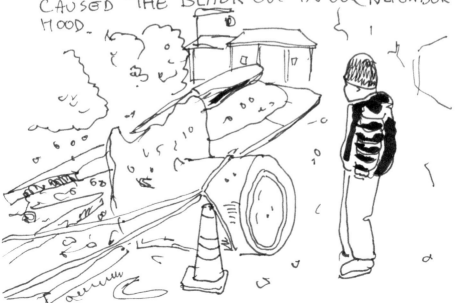

A FRIEND WROTE TO TELL ME SHE DREAMED LAST
NIGHT THAT I WAS SELLING MUD PIES SHAPED
LIKE GINGERBREAD MEN FROM A STAND
IN A SUBWAY STATION. I DON'T KNOW
WHY, BUT THAT GAVE ME A LIFT.

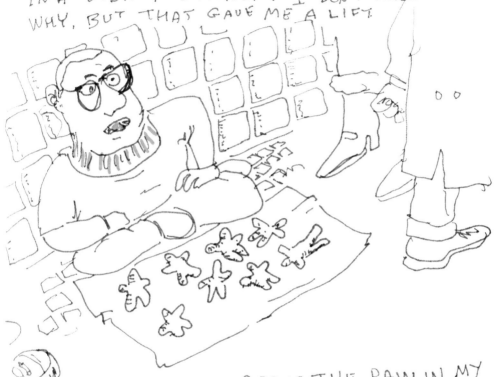

I'M WONDERING ABOUT THE PAIN IN MY
EAR, WHICH HAS COME BACK WITH A VENGEANCE
IN THE LAST FEW DAYS.   IT HAS BEEN
POSSIBLE OVER THESE   FIRST WEEKS
OF THERAPY TO   FORGET THAT
THE REASON FOR ALL   THESE
SHENANIGANS IS THAT I HAVE CANCER.
THE FOCUS HAS BEEN ON ALL THE GAMES-
MANSHIP OF THE TREATMENT. THE EAR
PAIN DISAPPEARED FOR AWHILE, BUT NOW
THAT ITS BACK, I HAVE TO DEAL
WITH THE IDEA OF BEING SICK AGAIN.

16 DAYS TO GO. IT WAS A VERY BAD RADIATION SESSION AND UNFORTUNATELY IT HAS TURNED ME AROUND. I'M KINDOF READY FOR ANYTHING NOW THAT WILL GET ME THROUGH THE NEXT 16 SESSIONS. SO KATHY WON THE BATTLE OF THE PADS ON THE NECK. I WALKED OUT OF THE HOSPITAL LOOKING LIKE A ~~SUR~~ SUR- VIVOR OF THE REIGN OF TERROR.

SHE IS ALSO GOING TO GIVE ME ATIVAN HALF AN HOUR BEFORE MY SESSION TO RELAX ME. I DON'T CARE NOW. I JUST WANT TO SURVIVE THESE SESSIONS. IT WAS TORTURE TO PUT THE MOUTHPIECE IN TODAY IT FELT LIKE MY JAW WAS BREAKING. ONCE THE MASK WAS ON MY MOUTH AND LIPS BEGAN TO SPASM AND QUIVER UNCON- TROLLABLY. I KNOW NOW TO BREATHE THROUGH MY NOSE BUT THE THICK MUCUS WAS COLLECTING TOO FAST FOR ME TO OVERCOME. ON TOP OF ALL THAT MY NECK SEEMS TO HAVE SWOLLEN MAKING THE MASK EVEN HARDER TO FORCE DOWN ONTO MY FACE. THE RAW SKIN ON MY NECK

W~~as~~ PARTICULARLY SORE AFTER THE SESSION BECAUSE OF THE PRESSURE FROM THE MASK.

OK! QUICK DUCT TAPE IT DOWN

THEY HAVE TO REALLY SCRUNCH IT DOWN ON MY HEAD TO MAKE THE MASK FIT.

NO PATCHES · THEN 25 mcg/h patch · THEN 37.5 mcg/h patches · NOW 50.0 mcg/h patches

I'VE BEEN GOING UP STEADILY WITH THE POWER OF MY PATCHES. I DON'T THINK IT'S DOING MUCH GOOD.

NOW I'M GETTING GRUMPY. I HATE TO TALK BECAUSE IT HURTS SO MUCH, BUT I SHOULDN'T RESENT IT WHEN PEOPLE WANT TO TALK TO ME. I SORT OF DO THOUGH. I SUSPECT THEY ARE TRYING TO TORTURE ME.

HOW ARE YOU FEELING, MATT? TALK!

I DON'T MIND PEOPLE TRYING TO FEED ME,
I APPRECIATE THE EFFORT. I JUST WISH
THEY WOULDN'T ASK ME WHAT TASTES
GOOD. **NOTHING TASTES GOOD.**
I HAVE NO SENSE OF TASTE. FOOD IS
SIMPLY MORE OR LESS TOLERABLE. WHAT
MAKES IT TOLERABLE IS THE AMOUNT
OF TIME IT TAKES TO SCRAPE ALONG
MY TONGUE AND THE ROOF OF MY MOUTH
AND THE BACK OF MY THROAT BEFORE I
CAN SWALLOW IT DOWN. THE LESS TIME,
THE MORE TOLERABLE. THE SMALLER THE
BITS OF SOLID MATERIAL IN THE FOOD, THE
LESS TIME, HENCE THE MORE TOLERABLE.

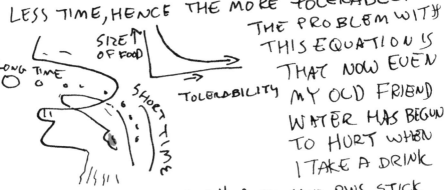

THE PROBLEM WITH
THIS EQUATION IS
THAT NOW EVEN
MY OLD FRIEND
WATER HAS BEGUN
TO HURT WHEN
I TAKE A DRINK
OF WATER ITS AS THOUGH A THOUSAND PINS STICK
INTO MY TONGUE AND THE INSIDE AND ROOF
OF MY MOUTH.

THIS AFTERNOON WE PASSED A DEAD PIGEON
ON THE WAY HOME FROM THE GROCERY STORE.

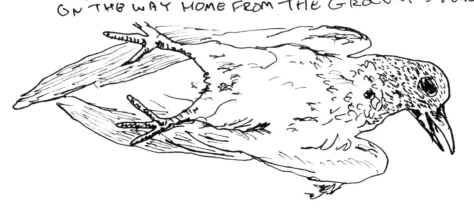

DAY 20

WHEN THIS DAY IS OVER I WILL BE $\frac{20}{35} = \frac{4}{7}$ OF THE WAY DONE. I WILL BE THROUGH FOUR WEEKS AND WILL HAVE THREE WEEKS TO GO. IT'S A SIGNIFICANT CHUNK, BUT GIVEN HOW BAD I'VE BEEN FEELING IN THE LAST FEW DAYS AND HOW THINGS HAVE BEEN RUNNING DOWN HILL, I DON'T FEEL VERY CONFIDENT ABOUT MY ABILITY TO COPE WITH WHAT IS COMING. THIS HAS BEEN A GREAT LESSON IN HUMILITY.

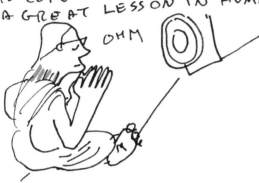

OHM

I HAVE BEEN USING A STAIR-WAY AS THE MET-APHOR TO DESCRIBE TO FRIENDS HOW EACH PROGRESSIVE DETERIORATION AFFECTS ME AND IS COPED WITH. I THINK THE METAPHOR IS DESIGNED MOSTLY TO ASSURE MY FRIENDS THAT I AM OK AND TO GIVE ME THE ILLUSION THAT I AM IN CON-TROL OF WHAT IS HAPPENING TO ME.

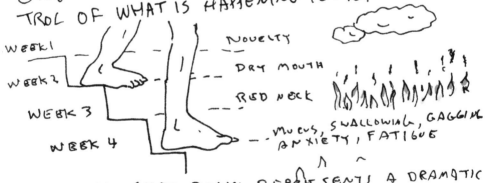

WEEK 1 — NOVELTY

WEEK 2 — DRY MOUTH

WEEK 3 — RED NECK

WEEK 4 — MUCUS, SWALLOWING, GAGGING, ANXIETY, FATIGUE

EACH NEW STEP DOWN REPRESENTS A DRAMATIC NEW SET OF PROBLEMS TO DEAL WITH AND THE END OF SOME ASPECT OF NORMALCY, SUCH AS EATING OR SPITTING, THAT WAS SO UNEXCEPTIONAL AS TO BE INVIS-IBLE, BUT THAT NOW SEEMS VITALLY IMPORTANT. EACH NEW SYMPTON, LIKE MY UNTOUCHABLE TONGUE, PRESENTS AN ALMOST CRUSHING NEW DIFFICULTY, ESPECIALLY WHEN I EXTRAPOLATE THE NEW PROBLEM OVER THE NEXT 2,3,4 OR 5 WEEKS: IT'S BAD NOW, HOW BAD CAN IT GET?

15

BUT AS THE NEW NORMAL SETS IN AFTER A FEW DAYS I SEEM TO ADAPT TO THE THE NEW LEVEL OF PAIN, OR MUCUS, OR BURN AND THE CONSEQUENTIAL NEW LEVEL OF MEDICATION OR EATING DIFFICULTY OR FATIGUE. I START TO FEEL A LITTLE MORE IN CONTROL AND A LITTLE BETTER IN MY NEW LOWER CIRCLE OF HELL. AND THAT'S SORT OF HAPPENING NOW. I'M ALL DOPED UP, I CAN'T GO FOR MORE THAN A MINUTE OR TWO WITHOUT SPITTING UP SOMETHING VILE, I CAN'T EAT ANYTHING FIRMER THAN A SCRAMBLED EGG. I CAN BARELY SPEAK ABOVE A WHISPER FOR MORE THAN A MINUTE BEFORE MY TONGUE FEELS AS IF IT IS ABOUT TO SNAP IN TWO AND FALL OUT OF MY MOUTH. BUT THAT'S OKAY. TONIGHT I CAN DEAL WITH THAT, TONIGHT.

SPIT MUCUS BURN

BEFORE THE ~~OTHER~~ SESSION TODAY KATHY AND JULIA SAT ME DOWN AND GAVE ME NEW MEDS AND A PEP TALK.

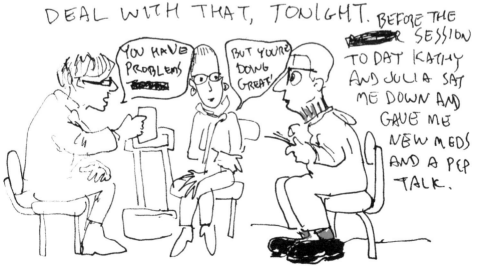

YOU HAVE PROBLEMS ~~....~~

BUT YOU'RE DOING GREAT!

HAD MY FIRST TWO MUCUS CUP SPILLS TODAY. IT'S NASTY GOOPY STUFF. STICKY AS GLUE, STRETCHY LIKE RUBBER CEMENT, SEMI-TRANSLUCENT, GLOSSY, WHITISH WITH YELLOW BLOBS AND PINK STRANDS FROM THE MAGIC MOUTH-WASH AND THE ROXICET.

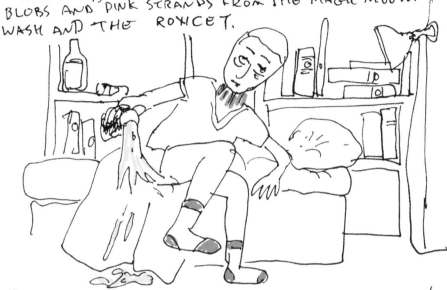

THIS MORNING AS I STUMBLED OUT OF BED, I SPILLED THE NIGHT'S WORTH OF COUGHED-UP SPUTUM. IT CLUNG TO THE COMFORTER LIKE GLUE.

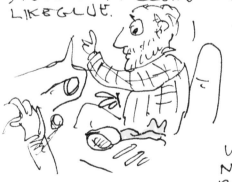

THEN THIS AFTERNOON ON THE DRIVE BACK FROM THE HOSPITAL I SPILLED THE DAY'S WORTH OF GOO ONTO BART'S PANTS. HE IMMEDIATELY WASHED ALL HIS CLOTHES, NOT JUST THE AFFECTED PANTS.

THESE BLOBS HAVE BEEN MOVING STEALTHILY & MOVING ABOUT THE APARTMENT FOR WEEKS. SOMETIMES THEY APPEAR TO ENGULF THE WADS OF TISSUE PAPER WITH TRULY DISGUSTING RESULTS.

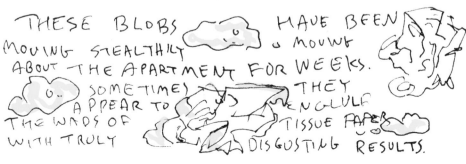

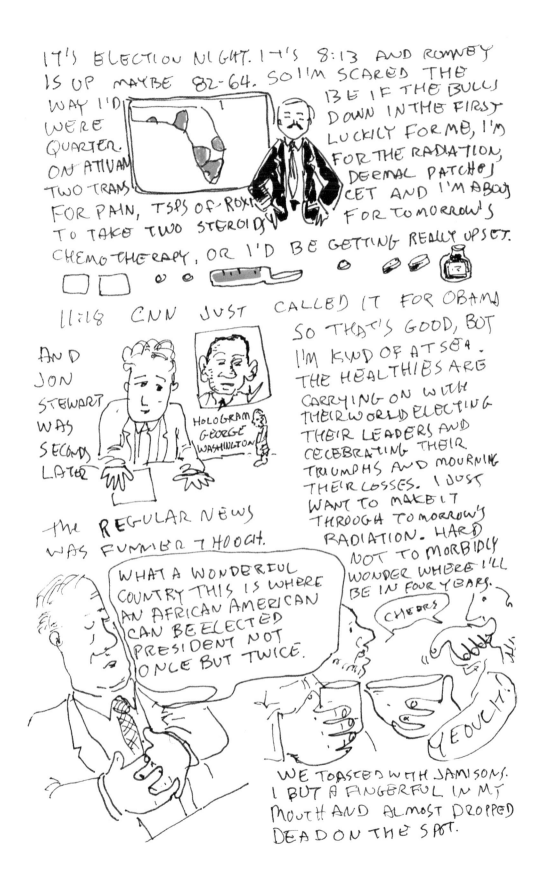

4 WEEKS OF THERAPY DOWN. 3 WEEKS TO GO.

14

DAYS TO GO.

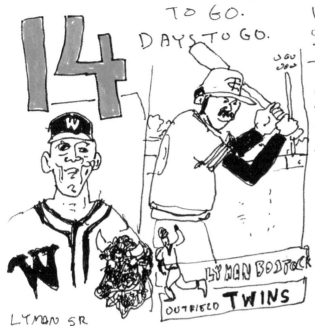

LYMAN SR PLAYED IN THE NEGRO LEAGUES FOR THE WINNIPEG BUFFALOES AND MANY OTHER TEAMS

OUTFIELD **TWINS**

LYMAN BOSTOCK

WE PARKED IN STALL **336** FOR SOME OBVIOUSLY DRUG RELATED REASON. AM MIXING UP NUMBERS AND LETTERS TODAY

THAT RANG A DISTANT MEMORY, LYMAN BOSTOCK! THE '70S JACK OF ALL TRADES BATTED 336 ONE YEAR BEFORE BEING MURDERED. WHY DOES THAT NUMBER STAY IN MY HEAD ALL THESE YEARS LATER, PARTICULARILY UNDER THESE CIRCUMSTANCES?

THIS MORNING NEITHER OF THE MEDICAL ONCOLOGISTS WAS THERE AND THE NURSE PRACTITIONER ACTED LIKE A FIRE WALL TO DISCOURAGE ANY OF JOSH'S GOOD IDEAS - TOPICAL PAIN MOUTHWASH THAT MAY BE MORE EFFECTIVE THAN THE ONE I'M ON.

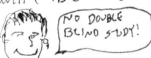

NO DOUBLE BLIND STUDY!

SALINE SOLUTION FOR DRINKING

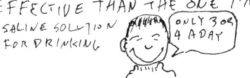

ONLY 3 OR 4 A DAY

BUT THE BIGGEST PROBLEM IS THAT SHE SAID DR. WIRTH WANTS TO SCHEDULE A FEEDING TUBE. I'M DOWN TO 180 LBS WHICH IS REALLY ONLY 2% DOWN FROM MY START WEIGHT. MY GONZO FATTENING UP, WHICH BRIEFLY BLEW ME UP TO 190 IS COMING BACK TO HAUNT ME. THREE POUNDS IN A WEEK ISN'T GOOD, BUT IT'S STILL WAY OFF FROM WHAT I THOUGHT WOULD BE THE CUT OFF WEIGHT FOR NEEDING THE TUBE.

190
180
170
160

165 lbs WOULD BE A 10% LOSS

0   1 WEEK 2   3   4   5 6

WHAT'S MOSTLY UPSETTING IS THAT I
THOUGHT WE HAD A DEAL; KEEP MY
WEIGHT UP, STAY OFF THE TUBE, I'M
GOING TO TRY TO REALLY FATTEN UP
FOR NEXT WEEK AND SEE WHAT THEY
SAY.

SO THIS IS
A NEW PATIENT:
PASSIVE-AGGRESSIVE
DUDE. MAYBE I CAN
BLUFF MY WAY
THROUGH.

NO, I CAN'T.
WHAT I AM
TRYING TO
SHIFT TO IS
EATING MATH

HOW DO YOU
LIKE THEM
APPLES?

TOWER
OF
ENSURE

AND AWAY FROM EATING LIKE A HUMAN
BEING. BEFORE, EVEN THOUGH I WAS TRYING
TO EAT TO NUMBER QUOTIENTS, 118 GRAMS OF
PROTEIN AND AROUND 2000 CALORIES, I WAS
REALLY ASSUMING—CORRECTLY, THAT I KNEW BY
HABIT OR SIGHT WHAT I NEED TO MAINTAIN
A STEADY WEIGHT.

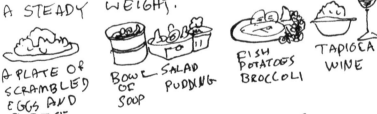

A PLATE OF
SCRAMBLED
EGGS AND
CHEESE

BOWL
OF
SOUP

SALAD
PUDDING

FISH
POTATOES
BROCCOLI

TAPIOCA
WINE

BUT NOW I CAN'T EAT ANYTHING STRONGER OR
RATHER THICKER THAN SOUP OR PUDDING.
MY GOAL IS 2000 PLUS CALORIES. 2500
WOULD BE NICE TO KEEP ME IN WHAT
I HOPE IS A RELATIVELY SAFE WEIGHT.
PROTEINS, I'M AFRAID ARE GOING TO HAVE
TO FEND FOR THEMSELVES.

NOW IT'S ALL ABOUT THE NUMBERS AND ALL THE BOTTLES AND TUBS HAVE LOTS OF NUMBERS ON THEM. IT'S HARD TO SWALLOW THE IDEA THAT THESE LITTLE CONTAINERS CAN MAKE ME KEEP MY PRESENT WEIGHT. BUT AFTER LAST NIGHT WHEN THE POLL NUMBER CRUNCHERS BEAT THE GUT TRUSTING PUNDITS. I'M ALL IN WITH THE MATH. IT'S MONEY BALL FOR NUTRITION, MONEY BELLY.

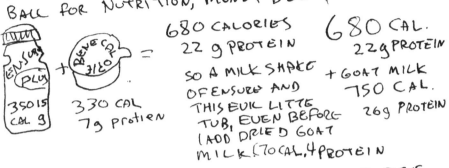

680 CALORIES
22 g PROTEIN

680 CAL.
22 g PROTEIN

ENSURE PLUS
35015 CAL 9

330 CAL
7g PROTIEN

SO A MILK SHAKE OF ENSURE AND THIS EVIL LITTE TUB, EVEN BEFORE I ADD DRIED GOAT MILK (70 CAL, 4 PROTEIN

+ GOAT MILK
750 CAL.
26 g PROTEIN

SO IF I JUST DRANK JUST 3 OF THESE GUT BOMBS I'M ALREADY AT 2250 CALORIES AND 78 GRAMS OF PROTEIN. THAT'S ALREADY SUPPOSEDLY ENOUGH TO KEEP MY WEIGHT UP. WITH A FEW TWEAKS HERE AND THERE IT WILL BE EASY, IT SEEMS TO GET TO THE 2500 - 3000 CALORIE LEVEL. WHETHER THAT'S HIGH ENOUGH IS ANOTHER QUESTION. BART HAS FOUND ON LINE DO-IT-YOURSELF CALORIE COUNTERS THAT SAY I HAVE TO EAT UP TO 5500 CALORIES JUST TO STAY EVEN. SO WHO KNOWS?

BEHIND ALL THE NUMBERS IS THE LOOMING POSSIBILITY THAT I SOON WON'T BE ABLE TO EAT OF DRINK ANYTHING AT ALL. EVERYTIME I BRUSH, GARGLE OR EAT THE INSIDE OF MY MOUTH FEELS LIKE HUNDREDS OF PIECES OF COTTAGE CHEESE ARE STUCK ON THE ROOF OF MY MOUTH AND TONGUE. THOSE ARE ALL PIECES OF SKIN SLOUGHING OFF MY MOUTH.

THE QUESTION OF WHETHER I'M IN CONTROL OR NOT IS DRIVING ME CRAZY. I CAN'T KEEP THOUGHTS TOGETHER FROM ONE MINUTE TO THE NEXT, SO I'M NOT EVEN SURE IF MY UNDERSTANDING OF WHAT IS HAPPENING IS CONSISTENT FROM DAY TO DAY.

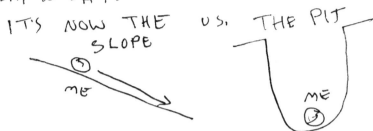

IT'S NOW THE SLOPE vs. THE PIT

ME

ME

IT'S NOT A STAIRWAY, IT'S A GRADUAL, LOGICAL ACCUMULATION OF SYMPTOMS I CAN DEAL WITH. OR IT'S EVERYTHING FALLING APART BAM! AND I'M SUDDENLY LOST. EVERY LITTLE THING THAT HAS BEEN GETTING WORSE DAY BY DAY REACHES A TIPPING POINT AND THEN IT'S ALL OVER.

NOTE TO SELF:

FROM NOW ON NO MORE LATE NIGHT RANTS ONLY LATE NIGHT DRAWINGS

1. THE RADIATION SUDDENLY TURNS INTO THE WATERBOARDING SESSION IT ALWAYS HAS FELT LIKE AND LITERALY I CAN'T BREATH ANY MORE.

2. THE REMAINING SKIN FALLS OFF THE REMAINS OF MY MOUTH AND NO AMOUNT OF PAIN RELIEF CAN MASK THE AGONY OF EATING.

3. THAT DOESN'T MATTER BECAUSE THE MUSCLES IN MY TONGUE AND THROAT BECOME SO STIFF AND UNRESPONSIVE THAT I SIMPLY CANNOT SWALLOW ANY KIND OF FOOD, LIQUID OR SOLID, AT ALL.

12:41 I HAVE TO STOP FINISHING THESE PAGES AM LATE AT NIGHT. I FORGET ALL THE IN- TERESTING THINGS I HAD TO SAY EARLIER AND ALL I HAVE LEFT IS AN INCOHERENT RANT.

THIS MORNING, THE FIRST DAY OF THE ALL NUMBERS ALL THE TIME DIET, I HAD THE 1400 SHAKE 350+330+70

+A 250CAL REGULAR ENSURE +8 TABLESPOONS OF HEAVY CREAM THE NUTRITIONIST WAS VERY IMPRESSED.

OF

"WATER THIS MORNING THAT WAS LIKE TRYING TO SWALLOW AN ANGRY CAT. NOW MY MOUTH IS OUT OF WHACK PH WISE ANYTHING WITHOUT SALT STINGS LIKE MAD.

YOU'RE MY HERO!

THE BACKSIDES OF MY TEETH FEEL LIKE MOSSY OLD DOCK PILINGS, FUZZY AND ROUGH WITH INCRUSTATIONS. THE GUMS BELOW ARE SENSITIVE AND SORE AND THE TEETH THEMSELVES ACHE NOW BUT I HAVEN'T YET HAD TO DEAL WITH ONE PREDICTED COMPLICATION: BROKEN AND BLOODY GUMS. I CAN STILL FLOSS BUT I CAN'T JUST PUSH THE ANGLE WHERE I WANTED IT TO GO.

NEWEST AREA OF CONCERN: THE BOTTOM OF THE TONGUE AND THE FLOOR OF THE MOUTH BOTH HAVE BECOME UNBELIEVABLY PAINFUL AND SENSITIVE IN THE LAST 48 HOURS

NECK INVENTORY— THIN AS TISSUE PAPER CRINKLY, VERY PAINFUL LOOKING RIGHT OR LEFT OR BEHIND IS A HIDEOUS EXPERIENCE.

NOW THE BACK OF MY EARS ARE DRYING OUT AND STARTING TO ITCH. CURIOUS AT FIRST, NOW A REAL ANNOYANCE.

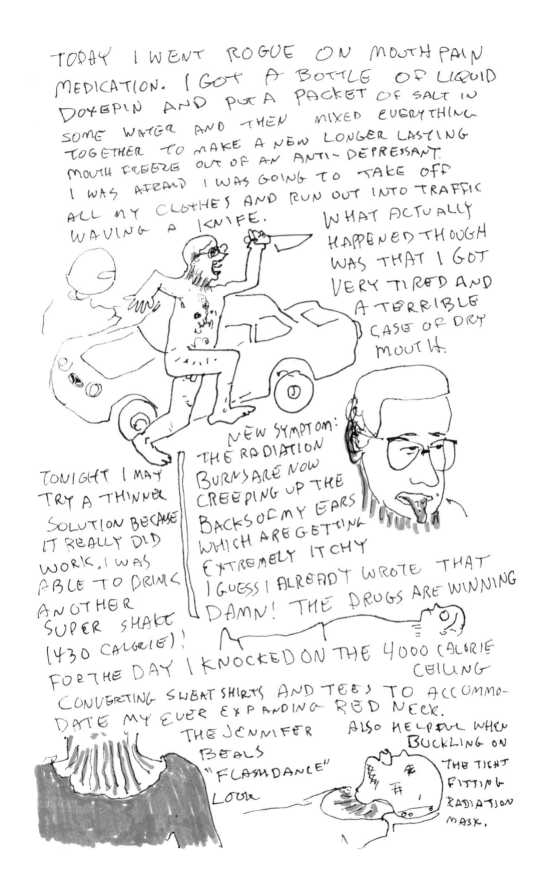

TODAY I WENT ROGUE ON MOUTH PAIN MEDICATION. I GOT A BOTTLE OF LIQUID DOXEPIN AND PUT A PACKET OF SALT IN SOME WATER AND THEN MIXED EVERYTHING TOGETHER TO MAKE A NEW LONGER LASTING MOUTH FREEZE OUT OF AN ANTI-DEPRESSANT. I WAS AFRAID I WAS GOING TO TAKE OFF ALL MY CLOTHES AND RUN OUT INTO TRAFFIC WAVING A KNIFE.

WHAT ACTUALLY HAPPENED THOUGH WAS THAT I GOT VERY TIRED AND A TERRIBLE CASE OF DRY MOUTH.

TONIGHT I MAY TRY A THINNER SOLUTION BECAUSE IT REALLY DID WORK. I WAS ABLE TO DRINK ANOTHER SUPER SHAKE (430 CALORIE)!

NEW SYMPTOM: THE RADIATION BURNS ARE NOW CREEPING UP THE BACKS OF MY EARS WHICH ARE GETTING EXTREMELY ITCHY I GUESS I ALREADY WROTE THAT DAMN! THE DRUGS ARE WINNING

FOR THE DAY I KNOCKED ON THE 4000 CALORIE CEILING

CONVERTING SWEATSHIRTS AND TEES TO ACCOMMODATE MY EVER EXPANDING RED NECK. THE JENNIFER BEALS "FLASHDANCE" LOOK

ALSO HELPFUL WHEN BUCKLING ON THE TIGHT FITTING RADIATION MASK.

IT IS LATE AT NIGHT AND I STILL HAVE
TWO MORE PAGES TO GO. I CAN'T SEEM
TO FIND THE TIME DURING THE DAY TO FINISH
MY ALLOTMENT OF PAGES.
WHICH IS A SHAME BECAUSE I'M A LOT MORE
COHERENT DURING THE DAY.
I'M SORT OF A WIND UP TOY.

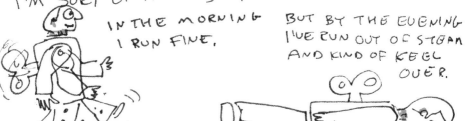

IN THE MORNING
I RUN FINE.

BUT BY THE EVENING
I'VE RUN OUT OF STEAM
AND KIND OF KEEL
OVER.

THE LARGER PATTERN REPEATS ITSELF
OVER THE COURSE OF THE WEEK.

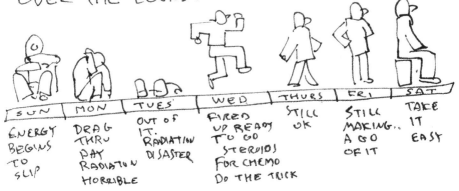

SUN	MON	TUES	WED	THURS	FRI	SAT
ENERGY BEGINS TO SLIP	DRAG THRU DAY RADIATION HORRIBLE	OUT OF IT. RADIATION DISASTER	FIRED UP READY TO GO STEROIDS FOR CHEMO DO THE TRICK	STILL OK	STILL MAKING.. A GO OF IT	TAKE IT EASY

BART GOES HOME   TOMORROW. IT WAS GOOD
TO HAVE HIM HERE.

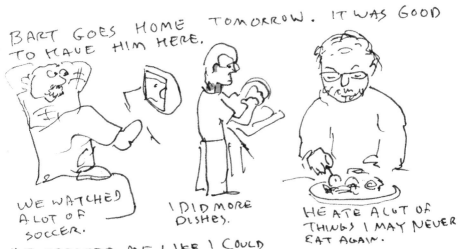

WE WATCHED
A LOT OF
SOCCER.

I DID MORE
DISHES.

HE ATE A LOT OF
THINGS I MAY NEVER
EAT AGAIN.

HE TREATED ME LIKE I COULD
TAKE CARE OF MYSELF. THAT WAS WONDERFUL.

IT'S TOO LATE TO THINK FOR ME NOW -
ALMOST MIDNIGHT, SO I WON'T ATTEMPT ANY
MORE THINKING AND RISKING ANOTHER
INCOHERENT RANT. THIS AFTERNOON BART
AND I WALKED OVER TO THE MASS
GENERAL HOSPITAL. IT'S NO MÜTTER
MUSEUM, BUT IT HAD SOME NICE STUFF.

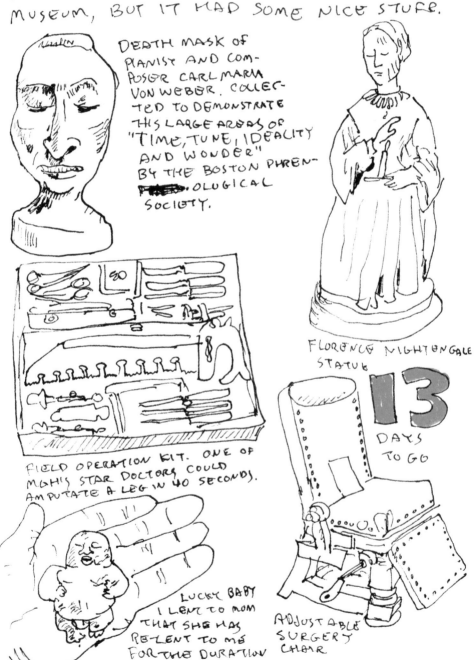

DEATH MASK OF
PIANIST AND COM-
POSER CARL MARIA
VON WEBER. COLLEC-
TED TO DEMONSTRATE
THIS LARGE AREAS OF
"TIME, TUNE, IDEALITY
AND WONDER"
BY THE BOSTON PHREN-
~~PHREN~~.OLOGICAL
SOCIETY.

FLORENCE NIGHTENGALE
STATUE

FIELD OPERATION KIT. ONE OF
MGH'S STAR DOCTORS COULD
AMPUTATE A LEG IN 40 SECONDS.

13
DAYS
TO GO

LUCKY BABY
I LENT TO MOM
THAT SHE HAS
RELENT TO ME
FOR THE DURATION
OF MY THERAPY.

ADJUSTABLE
SURGERY
CHAIR

ALL THAT CREAM IN THE SUPER SHAKES IS BRINGING BACK THE PHLEGM. I HOPE I'M NOT GOING TO GAG TOO BADLY IN RADIATION TODAY.

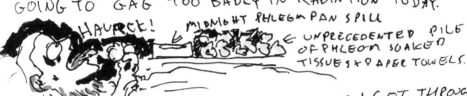

HAURCK!

MIDNIGHT PHLEGM PAN SPILL

UNPRECEDENTED PILE OF PHLEGM SOAKED TISSUES & PAPER TOWELS.

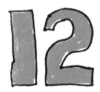

12
DAYS TO GO

AS IT TURNED OUT, I GOT THROUGH RADIATION IN "FINE" SHAPE, EVEN LYING THERE FOR AN EXTRA TEN MINUTES WHILE THEY WORKED OUT A GLITCH ON THEIR COMPUTER. I NOW HAVE AN EVEN MORE ELABORATE PRE-RADIATION RITUAL THAT CLEANS ME UP AND KNOCKS ME OUT.

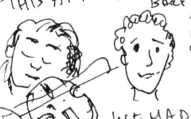

① BRUSH TEETH, TONGUE, ROOF OF MOUTH.

② GARGLE WITH ALKALOL

③ TAKE AN ATIVAN.

④ GARGLE WITH MAGIC MOUTH WASH.

⑤ TAKE TWO TSPS OF ROXICOT.

⑥ ONE LAST HACK AND SPIT.

THIS AFTERNOON I SAW JENNIE AND LESLEY BART AND JACK AT JUDY AND HUGHS

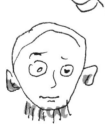

WE HAD A HUGE LUNCH THAT I ACTUALLY ENJOYED LOOKING AT AS I DRANK MY TWO BOTTLES OF ENSURE. I CELE-BRATED WITH A GRAPE AND A TINY PIECE OF SMOKED SALMON. I WAS STILL IN A DAZE FROM ALL THE RADIATION DRUGS, BUT I STILL HAD FUN.

I'M ALONE NOW FOR THE FIRST TIME IN WEEKS AND FOR THE LAST TIME DURING THERAPY. JACK TOOK BART TO THE AIRPORT A FEW HOURS AGO AND JUDE AND FLEURRY ARE MAKING TORTUROUSLY SLOW PROGRESS THROUGH THE BACKED UP ROADS FROM NEW YORK. I MAY HAVE ANOTHER HOUR ALONE. I DON'T HAVE MUCH I CAN DO NOW THOUGH BUT SIT STILL AND CLEAN MY TEETH AND DRINK 1500 CALORIE SHAKES.

BOSTON
SEATTLE
5 HOURS
3000 MILES.

NYC – BOSTON
200 MILES
7 PLUS HOURS

I FINALLY HAD A GOOD MEETING WITH DR. LIEBSCH THIS AFTERNOON. MY WEIGHT WAS UP A COUPLE OF POUNDS FROM WEDNESDAY THANKS TO MY SUPERSHAKES.

185
182
180

WED   FRI

FRI

AND MY MOUTH ULCERS WERE BETTER THAN LAST WEEK.

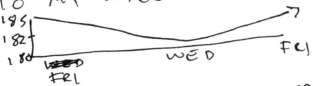

THIS IS A TRIBUTE TO GOOD ORAL CARE.

THIS IS ONLY A PARTIAL DEPICTION OF
ALL THE PILLS, WASHES, SYRUPS, POWDERS,
PADS AND DROPPERS I HAVE ACCUMULATED
IN THE PAST MONTH TO COPE WITH THE
EFFECTS OF THE RADIATION. DR. LIEBSCH
THINKS WE ARE DEEP ENOUGH INTO THE
PROCESS THAT THERE WILL NOT BE A
SUDDEN "NOSE DIVE" AHEAD THAT WILL
DRAMATICALLY IMPACT MY ABILITY TO
KEEP THINGS MOVING ALONG AND TO
KEEP ME OFF OF THE FEEDING TUBE.
I WAS PRETTY SUR- PRISED BY
HIS OPTIMISM.

I DON'T THINK THAT I'VE BEHAVED IN A PARTICULARLY EXEMPLARY WAY THROUGHOUT THE ILLNESS AND THERAPY - I AGREE WITH JON THAT NOBODY DOES WELL. PEOPLE - FRIENDS AND FAMILY TELL SICK PEOPLE THEY ARE DOING WELL OUT OF LOVE AND CONCERN AND TO ENCOURAGE THEM AND THAT'S FINE. WHAT STRIKES ME WHEN I'M SITTING IN THE WAITING ROOM AT THE PROTON CENTER WITH THE OTHER PATIENTS - NONE OF WHOM I THINK ARE DOING THAT WELL ON THE INSIDE, IS HOW WELL ALL OF THEM ARE DOING ON THE OUTSIDE - NOT THE SUPERFICIAL OUTSIDE, BUT THE BEHAVIORAL OUTSIDE. SICK PEOPLE ARE JUST ORDINARY PEOPLE DOING THE BEST THEY CAN. THAT'S USUALLY PRETTY GOOD. WE ARE PRETTY ADAPTIVE ANIMALS.

JUDE AND FLEURRY DROVE <u>NOV 10</u> UP YESTERDAY. I'VE BECOME SUCH A CREATURE OF HABIT THAT I HAD TO AD-JUST TO ALL THE NEW NOISE AND CHAOS. I COUNT UP MY CALORIES, I CLEAN MY TEETH, I COUGH UP SPITTLE, I MONITOR THE BURNS ON MY NECK, I RE-CALIBRATE MY PAIN MEDICATION. IT'S NOT MUCH OF A LIFE, BUT I'VE ADJUSTED TO IT. I FIND I AM TRYING TO PROTECT IT.

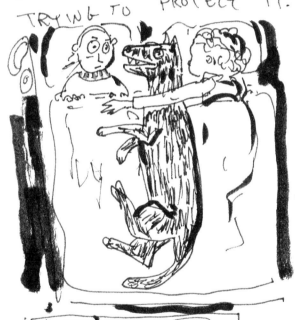

FLEURRY ENJOYS SLEEPING BETWEEN US THOUGH SHE RARELY SETTLES ON ONE SINGLE POSITION FOR THE ENTIRE NIGHT.

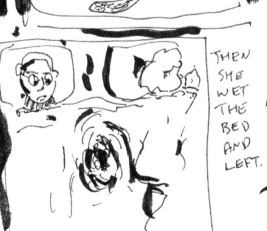

THEN SHE WET THE BED AND LEFT.

WOOF!

AT 3 AM SHE BEGAN TO BARK AT A CAT.

I NEED A NEW PROJECT TO WORRY
ABOUT. I'M WONDERING NOW IF I WILL
HAVE TIME TO MAKE LITTLE PRESENTS
FOR THE PEOPLE WHO HAVE HELPED ME.

DR. LIEBSCH L
DR. WIRTH L
DR. BENDAPUDI
KATHY L   KRMN L
PAUL L   TECH
  THE TECHS L

(WHAT A HIERARCHICAL
LIST! DRUGS HAVE
BLUNTED POLITICAL
CORRECTNESS INCLINATION

PROTON
GOD

JACKIE L
JULIA L

LIEBSCH

TONGUE
BUST

WIRTH

STOMACH TUBE

MASK
MAN

KATHY

DRINKER
JULIA

CHEMO
MAN

KRISTIN

WAITING
MAN

PAUL

MAN
ON SCALE
BENDAPUDI

MAN
WITH
PAPER
WORK

JACKIE

DON'T KNOW IF I HAVE ENOUGH EPOXY PLASTIC
FOR THIS, OR EVEN IF I DID WHETHER THIS WOULD
GO OVER TOO WELL WITH THE FOLKS HERE.
I KIND OF DOUBT IT, BUT THAT WON'T STOP ME.

OVER THE PAST FEW DAYS I'VE NOTICED AN ODD ECHOING IN PEOPLE'S VOICES OCCASIONALLY.

INCREDIBLY I KEPT TELLING MY SELF THE CAUSE WAS THE ACOUSTICS OF THE ROOM I WAS IN.

THIS MORNING IN THE TINY

H'MM DO-O I N L LAUN DRY REE N O O W E E ....

KITCHEN JUDE'S VOICE BEGAN SOUNDING LIKE IT WAS COMING FROM THE BOTTOM OF A WELL. SO NOW THERE'S SOMETHING NEW TO WORRY ABOUT — THOUGH HEARING PROBLEMS ARE PRETTY STANDARD FOR THIS THERAPY APPARENTLY.

MOM ARRIVED FROM CHICAGO WITH A TEETHING RING MY SISTER THOUGHT WOULD HELP. IT WASN'T TILL IT WAS ALREADY IN THAT IT OCCURRED TO ME THAT I ALREADY HAVE TEETH, SO RELIEF FROM GUM PAIN IS PROBABLY NOT MY HIGHEST PRI- ORITY. BUT I'LL TRY ANY THING, APPARENTLY.

BETTER?

MMGH

SATURDAY NIGHT AND ALL THE SYMPTOMS ARE STARTING TO PILE UP AGAIN. NOW I'M PREPARED FOR IT, BUT IT STILL FEELS TERRIBLE. I'M THREE DAYS INTO MY ALL NUMBERS DIET — 3970 CALORIES, 3840 CALORIES 3480 CALORIES. I SHOULD BE GETTING FATTER, BUT AT THIS RATE I MAY LOSE ALL DESIRE TO EAT BY THE END OF THE WEEKEND.

FOR SWALLOWING PRACTICE I ATE 120 CALORIES OF MIXED VEGETABLES AND PASTA BABY FOOD. IT HURT SO MUCH I HAD TO PACE AROUND THE ROOM AS I ATE TO SHOVEL EVERYTHING DOWN.

MOM AND JUDE AND FLEURRY WATCH AND TRY TO HELP AS I GO INTO MY WEEKEND TAILSPIN. I'M BEING KIND OF A JERK, BUT IT'S THE ONLY PLEASURE I HAVE LEFT. I THINK THEY UNDERSTAND. I MAKE THEM WATCH ME SPIT OUT MY THICK ROPEY PHLEGM.

THIS MORNING WE BEGGED OUT OF A STUDENT PRODUCTION OF THE MIKADO.

KIDS WE MIKADO WAS

WHEN WE WERE THOUGHT THE THE AVOCADO.

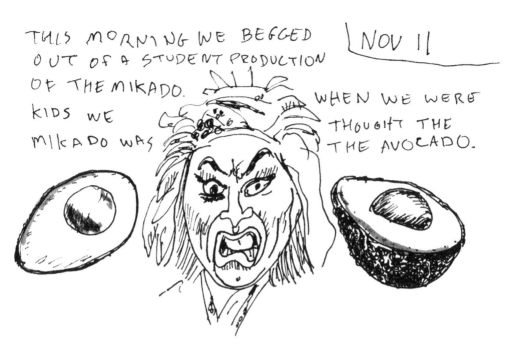

I HATE TO DROP OUT OF COMMITMENTS, PARTIALLY BECAUSE I WORRY ABOUT ALL SIGNALS THAT THINGS ARE FINALLY FOR SURE FALLING APART FOR GOOD, BUT I REALLY DID FEEL BAD THIS MORNING NOW I FEEL BETTER.

I FELT BETTER LAST NIGHT TOO WHEN I WORKED ON THE NINE LITTLE FIGURES FOR THE DOCTORS AND STAFF WHO HAVE BEEN HELPING ME. SOMEHOW FOCUSING ON SOMETHING SPECIFIC SHORT-CIRCUITS THE PAIN CONNECTIONS.

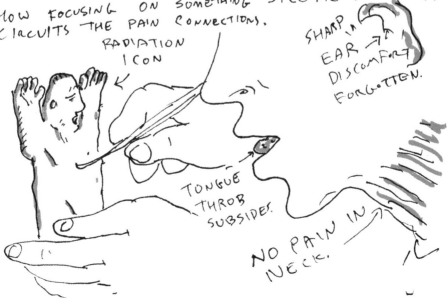

RADIATION ICON

SHARP EAR DISCOMFORT FORGOTTEN.

TONGUE THROB SUBSIDES.

NO PAIN IN NECK.

JUDE IS LOOKING FOR POEMS TO PASS ON TO HER GRAD STUDENTS. I WAS ALWAYS FOND OF THAT STEM WINDER BY CHARLES BUKOWSKI "THE LAUGHING HEART" BECAUSE IT HAS GOOD SPIRIT RAISING LINES FOR YOUNG ARTISTS.

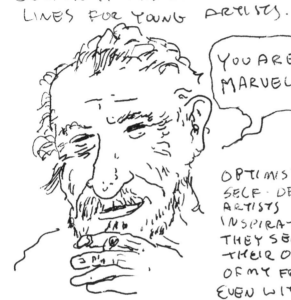

YOU ARE MARVELOUS —

OPTIMISTIC BUT SELF-DESTRUCTIVE ARTISTS ARE VERY INSPIRATIONAL FIGURES THEY SEEM TO DESERVE THEIR OPINIONS, ONE OF MY FRIENDS SAYS THAT, EVEN WITH CANCER I PROBABLY LIVE A HEALTHIER LIFE THAN BUKOWSKI OR BURROUGHS EVER DID. ITS TRUE. I'M NOT MUCH OF A TRAGIC POET. AN ACCIDENTAL TOUCH OF CANCER, A CHOPPED THUMB, BORDERLINE HYPER TENSION IS ABOUT ALL I HAVE TO OFFER.

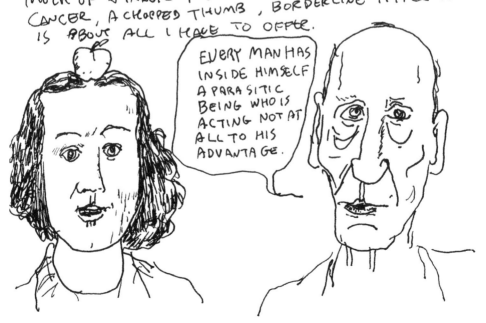

EVERY MAN HAS INSIDE HIMSELF A PARASITIC BEING WHO IS ACTING NOT AT ALL TO HIS ADVANTAGE.

IT'S HARD TO REMEMBER, GIVEN HOW PRE-OCCUPYING ALL THE RADIATION SYMPTOMS HAVE BEEN THAT THEY ARE REALLY ONLY THE TIP OF THE ICEBERG.

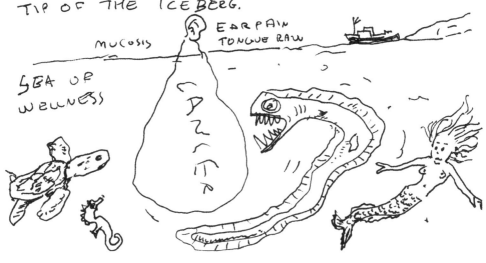

EARPAIN TONGUE RAW

MUCOSIS

CANCER

SEA OF WELLNESS

MY FRIEND DAVID CALLED TODAY FROM A PLAYGROUND IN BROOKLYN WHILE HE WAS WATCHING HIS DAUGHTER. SOMEHOW THE COMBINATION OF RECITING MY SYMPTOMS AND PROSPECTS OVER THE SOUNDS OF SHRIEKING KIDS PUT ME BACK IN A BIT OF OF A SENTIMENTAL SPIRAL.

WHEE!

WHAT NEXT?

THEN WE START LOOKING FOR SOME-THING TO CURE THE TUMORS IN THE LUNGS.

THOSE NASTY TUMORS IN THE LUNGS- SITTING THERE CALMLY WHILE THIS STORM IN MY HEAD AND NECK IS RAGING JUST A FEW INCHES ABOVE THEM. WAITING, BIDING THEIR TIME, PRE-PARED TO STRIKE AT A MOMENT'S NOTICE.

TROJAN HORSE

IN LUNGS

TONIGHT MY MOTHER BROUGHT UP
THE MATTER OF THE DENTIST AGAIN
MY DENTIST IS A GREAT DENTIST. HE

LOVES THE LATEST DENTIST TECHNOLOGY.
HE USES 3-D MILLING MACHINES IN HIS OFFICE
THAT ARE CONNECTED WIRELESSLY TO A SCANNER
TO MAKE CERAMIC INLAYS FOR INFECTED TEETH.
HE LOVES TO THINK ABOUT TEETH AND HE
LOVES TO TALK ABOUT TEETH.

BUT HE NEVER FOUND THE TUMOR AT
THE BASE OF MY TONGUE IN ALL THOSE
YEARS, AND HE NEVER FELT THE SWOLLEN
NODES IN MY NECK WHEN THEY POPPED
UP MORE RECENTLY. SHOULD HE HAVE
FOUND THEM? PROBABLY NOT. HE WOULD
HAVE HAD TO REACH SO
FAR DOWN MY THROAT
TO FIND THE TUMOR IN
THE EARLY YEARS THAT
I WOULD HAVE GAGGED.
NOT THE WAY YOU WANT TO TREAT
YOUR PATIENTS BY AND LARGE.
BUT MY MOTHER SAYS HER DENTIST
ALWAYS FEELS FOR LUMPS IN THE NECK
AND WOULD HAVE FOUND SOME-
THING.

AHA!

THERE!
OBVIOUS!

NOW, OF COURSE
EVERYONE WHO
LOOKS IN MY MOUTH
SEES EVERYTHING
RIGHT AWAY
IT'S A SMALL THING
TO MISS. I WONDER
WHAT MY LIFE WOULD HAVE BEEN LIKE IF IT HADN'T
BEEN MISSED FOR ALL THOSE YEARS.

ALMOST IMMEDIATELY IN STALL 4, THAT'S LOU GEHRIG'S NUMBER. THAT'S A REAL ROLE MODEL. GREAT PLAYER, OVER-SHADOWED BY BABE RUTH, DIED YOUNG OF HIS OWN DISEASE.

BUT JUDE PARKED HALF IN THE 5 STALL.

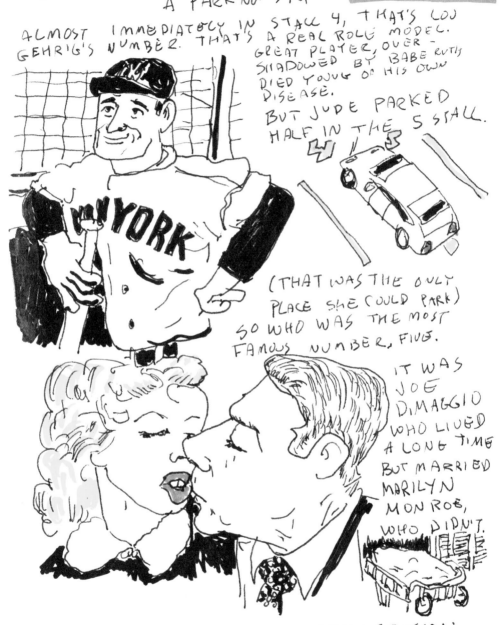

(THAT WAS THE ONLY PLACE SHE COULD PARK) SO WHO WAS THE MOST FAMOUS NUMBER, FIVE.

IT WAS JOE DIMAGGIO WHO LIVED A LONG TIME BUT MARRIED MARILYN MONROE, WHO DIDN'T.

IT WAS A PRETTY ROUGH RADIATION SESSION. I HAVE A VERY ELABORATE RITUAL NOW THAT WORKS PRETTY WELL, BRUSHING, SPITTING, SWIGS OF PAIN KILLERS AND ANT-ANXIETY MEDS. I KIND OF GO THROUGH IN A DAZE NOW. SHOULDN'T HAVE GIVEN THEM A 40 YEAR OLD NATIONAL LAMPOON CD THOUGH. PC COMEDY STANDARDS HAVE CHANGED OVER THE YEARS. I LIKE YOU   MR. ROGERS! YOU TOUCHED MY KID!

THIS AFTERNOON OUR COUSINS TODD AND SUE AND THEIR DAUGHTER AVA CAME TO VISIT. THEY LIVE ON MARTHA'S VINEYARD WHERE FOR YEARS TODD BUILT BEAUTIFUL WOODEN BOATS AND HOUSES.

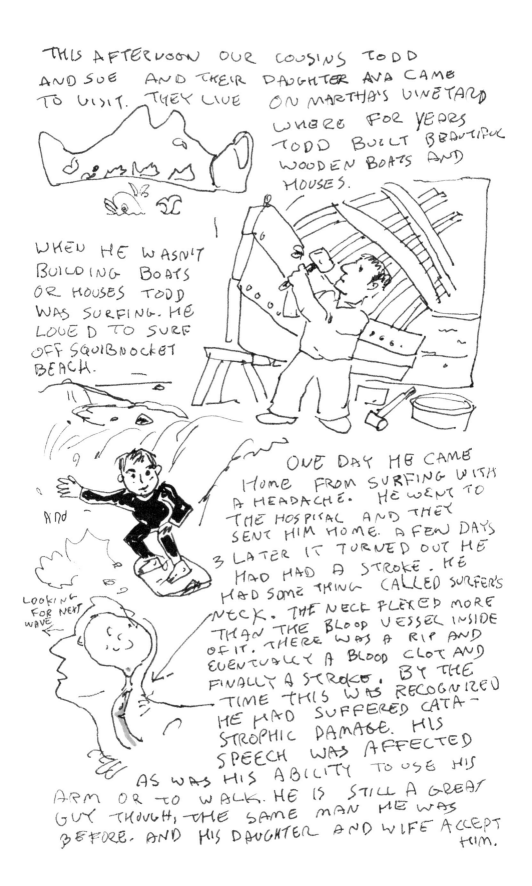

WHEN HE WASN'T BUILDING BOATS OR HOUSES TODD WAS SURFING. HE LOVED TO SURF OFF SQUIBNOCKET BEACH.

AND

LOOKING FOR NEXT WAVE ←

ONE DAY HE CAME HOME FROM SURFING WITH A HEADACHE. HE WENT TO THE HOSPITAL AND THEY SENT HIM HOME. A FEW DAYS LATER IT TURNED OUT HE HAD HAD A STROKE. HE HAD SOMETHING CALLED SURFER'S NECK. THE NECK FLEXED MORE THAN THE BLOOD VESSEL INSIDE OF IT. THERE WAS A RIP AND EVENTUALLY A BLOOD CLOT AND FINALLY A STROKE. BY THE TIME THIS WAS RECOGNIZED HE HAD SUFFERED CATA-STROPHIC DAMAGE. HIS SPEECH WAS AFFECTED AS WAS HIS ABILITY TO USE HIS ARM OR TO WALK. HE IS STILL A GREAT GUY THOUGH, THE SAME MAN HE WAS BEFORE. AND HIS DAUGHTER AND WIFE ACCEPT HIM.

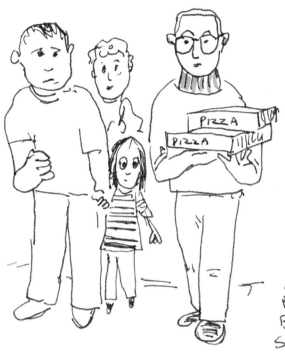

I WENT TO PICK UP PIZZAS BEFORE THEY SHOWED UP AND TODD WALKED OVER WITH AVA AND MY MOTHER TO MEET ME. IT WAS WONDERFUL TO SEE HIM. NEITHER OF US COULD TALK MUCH. FOR SEVEN YEARS. THIS WAS A POINT OF DISCOMFORT WITH TODD. BUT NOW, HE CAN SPEAK BETTER THAN I CAN.

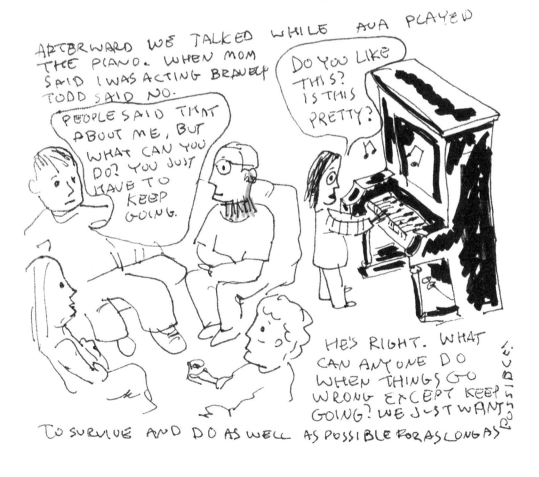

AFTERWARD WE TALKED WHILE AVA PLAYED THE PIANO. WHEN MOM SAID I WAS ACTING BRAVELY TODD SAID NO.

PEOPLE SAID THAT ABOUT ME, BUT WHAT CAN YOU DO? YOU JUST HAVE TO KEEP GOING.

DO YOU LIKE THIS? IS THIS PRETTY?

HE'S RIGHT. WHAT CAN ANYONE DO WHEN THINGS GO WRONG EXCEPT KEEP GOING? WE JUST WANT TO SURVIVE AND DO AS WELL AS POSSIBLE FOR AS LONG AS POSSIBLE.

THIS AFTERNOON I WEIGHED MYSELF TO GLOAT OVER MY FIVE DAYS OF HIGH CALORIE EATING. I'D ALREADY GONE UP A COUPLE OF POUNDS AND I WAS COUNTING ON ANOTHER BUMP UP BUT I WAS WRONG. MY WEIGHT WAS DOWN ABOUT FIVE POUNDS TO 177 SOMETHING. DAMN! ALL THOSE AWFUL SHAKES AND I'M STILL SLIDING BACKWARDS. KATHY SAYS NOT TO WORRY AND JOSH SAYS THAT'S WATER WEIGHT LOSS NOT CALORIE WEIGHT LOSS.

AND MAYBE, IN FACT, CALORIES DON'T EVEN MATTER.

BUT STILL CALORIES ARE THE ONLY THING I CAN CONTROL. SO I DOUBLED DOWN. TODAY I BROKE THROUGH THE 4000 CALORIE BARRIER **4120!** A SUPER SHAKE, A SHAKE, A MEDIUM SEMI-MEDIUM SHAKE, SOME EGGS AND MUSHROOMS AND EVEN A PLATE OR TEENY TINY BITS OF STEAK.

STEAK! MOM BOUGHT HERSELF A STEAK AND I DON'T THINK SHE CAN BELIEVE THAT THERE IS ANY SOURCE OR PROTIEN AS EFFICIENT, SO I ATE IT. I FEEL LIKE I'M PREPARING A LEGAL DEFENSE FOR MY FEEDING TUBE APPEAL. "BUT I ATE STEAK ON MONDAY." "BUT I ATE 4000 CALORIES A DAY!" WHETHER OR NOT THAT ACTUALLY HAS ANYTHING TO DO WITH ACTUAL HEALTHY EATING.

WHEN I WAS YOUNG I ATTEMPTED TO CURRY FAVOR AND ATTENTION IN MY BIG FAMILY BY ACTING LIKE A KIND OF IN-HOUSE ELF.

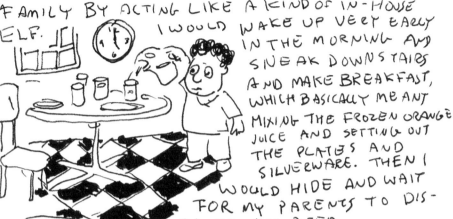

I WOULD WAKE UP VERY EARLY IN THE MORNING AND SNEAK DOWNSTAIRS AND MAKE BREAKFAST, WHICH BASICALLY MEANT MIXING THE FROZEN ORANGE JUICE AND SETTING OUT THE PLATES AND SILVERWARE. THEN I WOULD HIDE AND WAIT FOR MY PARENTS TO DIS- COVER MY DEED.

I HAVE NO IDEA. MUST HAVE BEEN ONE OF THE KIDS. MUST HAVE BEEN MATT!

WHO COULD HAVE DONE THIS?

I ALSO LOVED TO WAKE UP EARLY SO I COULD GET THE CHICAGO SUN-TIMES ROLLED UP IN A TUBE ON THE FRONT LAWN.

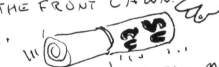

THOSE WERE THE FIRST GREAT MOMENTS OF DRAMA IN MY LIFE, WAITING TO FIND OUT AS I CAREFULLY ROLLED THE RUBBER BAND OFF THE PAPER, IF THE CUBS OR SOX HAD WON THE DAY BEFORE.

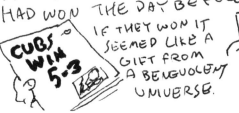

CUBS WIN 5-3

IF THEY WON IT SEEMED LIKE A GIFT FROM A BENEVOLENT UNIVERSE.

SOX SWEPT 3-2, 9-7

IF THEY LOST, IT CONFIRMED MY PESSIMISTIC ASSUMPTIONS ABOUT FATE. EITHER WAY, IT WAS EXCITING.

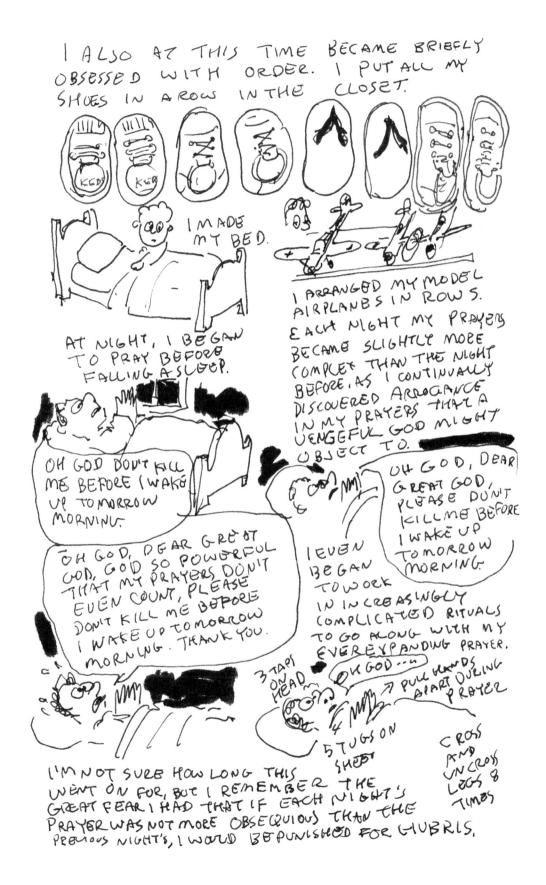

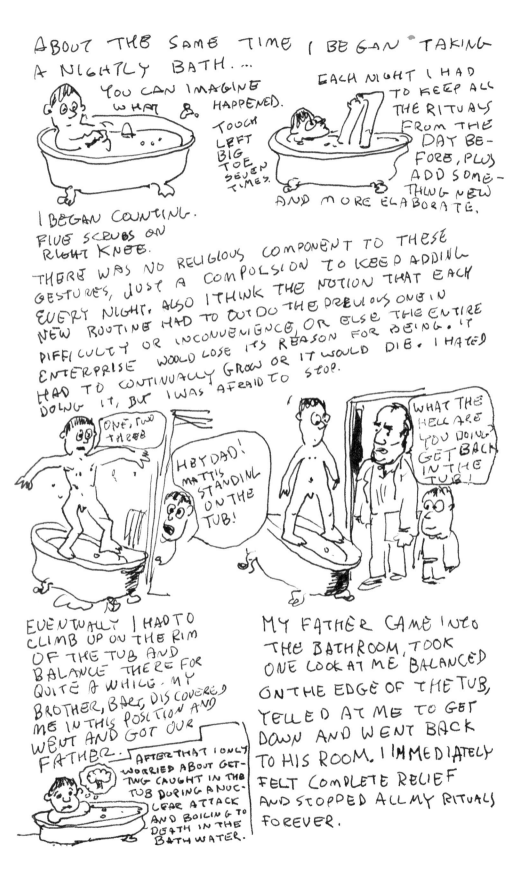

ABOUT THE SAME TIME I BEGAN TAKING A NIGHTLY BATH....

YOU CAN IMAGINE WHAT HAPPENED.

TOUCH LEFT BIG TOE SEVEN TIMES.

EACH NIGHT I HAD TO KEEP ALL THE RITUALS FROM THE DAY BEFORE, PLUS ADD SOMETHING NEW AND MORE ELABORATE.

I BEGAN COUNTING. FIVE SCRUBS ON RIGHT KNEE.

THERE WAS NO RELIGIOUS COMPONENT TO THESE GESTURES, JUST A COMPULSION TO KEEP ADDING EVERY NIGHT. ALSO I THINK THE NOTION THAT EACH NEW ROUTINE HAD TO OUTDO THE PREVIOUS ONE IN DIFFICULTY OR INCONVENIENCE, OR ELSE THE ENTIRE ENTERPRISE WOULD LOSE ITS REASON FOR BEING. IT HAD TO CONTINUALLY GROW OR IT WOULD DIE. I HATED DOING IT, BUT I WAS AFRAID TO STOP.

ONE, TWO, THREE

HEY DAD! MATT IS STANDING ON THE TUB!

WHAT THE HELL ARE YOU DOING? GET BACK IN THE TUB!

EVENTUALLY I HAD TO CLIMB UP ON THE RIM OF THE TUB AND BALANCE THERE FOR QUITE A WHILE. MY BROTHER, BART, DISCOVERED ME IN THIS POSITION AND WENT AND GOT OUR FATHER.

AFTER THAT I ONLY WORRIED ABOUT GETTING CAUGHT IN THE TUB DURING A NUCLEAR ATTACK AND BOILING TO DEATH IN THE BATH WATER.

MY FATHER CAME INTO THE BATHROOM, TOOK ONE LOOK AT ME BALANCED ON THE EDGE OF THE TUB, YELLED AT ME TO GET DOWN AND WENT BACK TO HIS ROOM. I IMMEDIATELY FELT COMPLETE RELIEF AND STOPPED ALL MY RITUALS FOREVER.

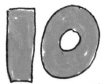 **MORE DAYS TO GO. THE FINAL COUNTDOWN BEGINS.**

MY JEWISH EDUCATION WAS SPOTTY. I STUDIED FOR MY BAR MITZVAH, BUT MY GRANDFATHER HAD A STROKE TWO WEEKS BEFORE SO WE CANCELLED IT. HE WAS THE ONLY ONE WHO CARED. HE WAS BORN IN THE TOWN OF DOKSHITZ ON THE FIFTH NIGHT OF CHANNUKAH LATE IN THE NINETEETH CENTURY.

ONCE A COUSIN WISHED HIM A MERRY CHRISTMAS (IT HAPPENED TO BE CHRISTMAS) GRANDPA SAM BECAME VERY UPSET.

CALM DOWN GRANDPA

MERRY CHRISTMAS!? MERRY CHRISTMAS?! MILLIONS OF JEWS WERE MURDERED ON CHRISTMAS!

I SUPPOSE BACK IN DOKSHITZ THERE PROBABLY WERE POGROMS AGAINST THE JEWS ON CHISTMAS.

I GUESS THEY COULD HAVE USED A GOLEM IN DOKSHITZ.

INSTEAD I HAD A CONFIRMATION CEREMONY AT OUR LOCAL SYNAGOGUE IN CHICAGO WHEN I TURNED FIFTEEN. I HAD TO GO TO LOTS OF SERVICES.

THERE WAS A LITTLE TOO MUCH OF MY CHILDHOOD OBESSIVE PRAYERS IN THE LITURGY.

WE ARE UNWORTHY

THE SYNAGOGUE KAM ISAIAH ISRAEL IS A FEW BLOCKS FROM WHERE I GREW UP AND I GOT MUGGED DOZENS OF TIMES.

ABOUT TEN YEARS AGO A YOUNG POLITICIAN AND HIS FAMILY MOVED IN ACROSS THE STREET.

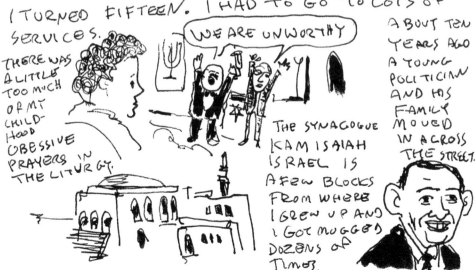

DAY 26 AFTER YESTERDAY'S | NOV 19 | DIFFICULT RADIATION TODAY'S STEROID-FUELED ONE WAS AN OLD FASHIONED BREEZE. I EVEN NODDED OFF A TIME OR TWO. I AM REDDER AND SORER THAN EVER, AND THIS ALMOST ALL LIQUID DIET IS NOT A LOT OF FUN, BUT I'M MORE HOPEFUL NOW THAT IT CAN'T GET MUCH WORSE. THE DOCTORS THOUGH REFUSE TO PLAY ALONG. THEY SUBSCRIBE TO THE "NOSE DIVE" THEORY, WHEREBY EVERYTHING IS FINE ONE DAY AND THEN THE NEXT I AM TOTALLY INCAPACITATED. THAT'S WHY THE FEEDING TUBE IS STILL SCHEDULED TO BE PUT IN ON THE DAY AFTER THANKSGIVING, WITH ONLY THREE MORE RADIATIONS ON THE SCHEDULE.

NOSE DIVE

ROAD TO WELLNESS

INCAPACITY

AT THE MEETINGS THIS MORNING THERE WAS GENERAL APPLAUSE FOR MY 4000 CALORIES A DAY NUMBERS DIET, BUT THEY ARE KEEPING THE STOMACH TUBE, WHICH THEY CALL A G TUBE ON THE BOOKS. THE MUCOSIS IS GETTING WORSE.

SCHEMATIC OF MOUTH INDICATING LEVEL OF MUCOSIS.

THE GOO IS EVERYWHERE AND IT SOMETIMES TAKES TWO OR THREE SWIGS OF MAGIC MOUTHWASH JUST TO GET THROUGH A BOTTLE OF ENSURE. SO THEY MAY HAVE A POINT. I MAY BE HEADING FOR A NOSE DIVE.

THE TOPIC OF DOPE PIN CAME UP. DR. BENDAPUDI TACTFULLY SPECULATED THAT I MIGHT HAVE "BLACK MARKET" ACCESS TO SOME. THEY'RE ON TO THE FREEDMAN BROTHERS I THINK.

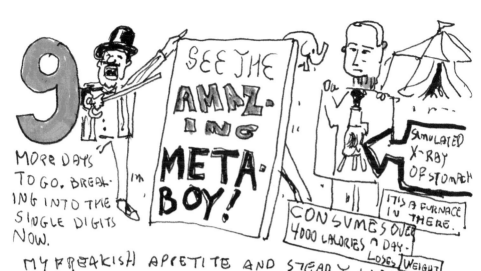

9

SEE THE AMAZ-ING META-BOY!

SIMULATED X-RAY OF STOMACH

IT'S A FURNACE IN THERE.

CONSUMES OVER 4000 CALORIES A DAY — LOSES WEIGHT

MORE DAYS TO GO. BREAKING INTO THE SINGLE DIGITS NOW.

MY FREAKISH APPETITE AND STEADY WEIGHT HAS AMUSED MY FRIENDS AND PLEASED ME FOR YEARS. I ALMOST NEVER GET FULL, AND I STAY AT ABOUT 185 POUNDS NO MATTER WHAT. NOW I'M POURING IN THE CALORIES AND AM SLOWLY DRIFTING BACKWARDS. 183-186-190-184↓177/182-177-179 (STUPIDLY TRIED TO FATTEN UP EARLIER) AT LEAST NOW I HAVE SCIENCE BACKING UP WHAT EVERYONE ALREADY KNEW. I'M THE ORIGINAL STARVING ARTIST.

BACK IN CHEMO. MY VEINS MUST BE GETTING TIRED. FOR THE SECOND WEEK IN A ROW THE FIRST VEIN WE POKED INTO FAILED AND WE HAD TO GO LOOKING FOR A SECOND SITE. THIS TIME WE SETTLED ON A BIG BLUE VEIN ON THE BACK OF MY HAND. THE INFUSION STUNG AT FIRST BUT NOW I'M USED TO IT. THEY WANT ME TO RAISE MY PAIN PATCHES BY ANOTHER 50% BUT I'M RESISTING AGAIN.

META BOY

I THINK THE NEXT COUPLE OF DAYS WILL BE THE TEST. IF I CAN GET THROUGH THEM WITH ONLY MINOR DETERIORATION I SHOULD BE GOOD. IF NOT, I'D LOOKING AT THE G-TUBE OR WORSE INTERRUPTION.

LOWERED EXPECTATIONS HAVE ALWAYS SERVED ME WELL. NOW I'M AT THE TIPPING-POINT (AGAIN!) AND I NEED TO KEEP MY EYES DOWN RIGHT ON MY TOES AND GO ONE BOTTLE OF ENSURE, ONE SWIG OF MAGIC MOUTH WASH, ONE NEW DERMAL PATCH-AT A TIME. IT DOESN'T HELP TO BE TOLD I'M DOING GREAT. (WHO BUT A FIVE YEAR OLD SHOULD BE CELEBRATED FOR FINISHING THEIR DINNER?)

YOU ATE ALL YOUR SOUP! GREAT!

EVERY TIME I HEAR HOW WELL I'M DOING I THINK PEOPLE EXPECT ME TO DO WELL, AND NO ONE DOES WELL AT THIS. YOU JUST SURVIVE IT. OR YOU DON'T, ACTUALLY WHEN THE CHICAGO BULLS WERE ON THEIR GREAT RUN IN THE NINETIES, I USUALLY KEPT THE SOUND OFF DURING THE PLAYOFF GAMES BECAUSE THE ANNOUNCERS WOULD ALWAYS BEGIN THE GAME BY SAYING THE BULLS WERE THE GREATEST TEAM EVER. THEN WHEN THE GAME TURNED OUT TO BE CLOSE, AS THEY USUALLY WERE, ALL THEY WOULD SAY WAS WHAT A GREAT UPSET IT WOULD BE IF THE BULLS FINALLY LOST. THEY ALMOST NEVER DID, BUT I COULDN'T STAND THE RAISED EXPECTATIONS.

I WONDER IF DONALD PATRAEUS, SUBJECT OF THE LATEST WASHINGTON D.C. SEX SCANDAL, WORRIES ABOUT RAISED EXPECTATIONS. I SUPPOSE NOT. THAT'S NOT A TOWN WHERE THEY WORRY ABOUT THAT. THAT'S HOW THEY GET WHERE THEY GET AND WHY EVERYONE SEEMS TO ENJOY IT SO MUCH WHEN THEY FAIL SO SPECTACULARLY. DONALD PATRAEUS WOULDN'T NEED ONE PAIN PATCH TO GET THROUGH THIS. HE'D PROBABLY SHAVE HIS NECK WITH A RAZOR LIKE MY OLD PROFESSOR SCHMIDT TO SPEED THE HEALING PROCESS. OF COURSE, IT TURNED OUT HE DID NEED A CHEERING SQUAD TO KEEP HIM MOTIVATED SO MAYBE HE'S NOT

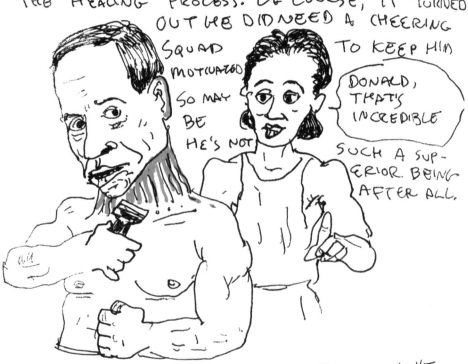

DONALD, THAT'S INCREDIBLE

SUCH A SUPERIOR BEING AFTER ALL.

I DON'T KNOW WHY I HAVE TO FIGHT EVERY ESCALATION IN THE PAIN MANAGEMENT OF THIS THERAPY. I'M HAPPY EACH TIME THE MEDS GO UP, OR AT LEAST I APPRECIATE THE RELATIVE LACK OF PAIN. BUT I DO KEEP RESISTING. I'M AFRAID IF I DIDN'T I WOULDN'T KNOW IF I WAS REALLY STILL ME IN THE MIDDLE OF ALL THIS. IT'S A GOOD THING I'M SURROUNDED BY MUCH MORE SENSIBLE PEOPLE.

IN MOUTH. EVEN AS I GET MORE USED TO MY SYMPTOMS AND MORE METHODICAL IN MY PREPARATIONS TO MY TREATMENTS, EVERYTHING CONTINUES TO GET WORSE. IT'S SORT OF A RACE FOR ENLIGHTEMENT IN WHICH THEY KEEP MOVING THE FINISH LINE BACKWARDS. THE QUESTION IS DO I HAVE ENOUGH PAIN RELIEVERS AND PATCHES AND MAGIC MOUTH WASH TO KEEP ME SWALLOWING AND GET ME OVER THE FINISH LINE? I THINK I DO. BUT IT COULD BE CLOSE. I'M GOING TO EXPERIMENT WITH JOSH'S SUPER ANTI-ANXIETY MOUTHWASH. I'M GOING THROUGH A BOTTLE OF MAGIC MOUTHWASH A DAY NOW.

I PARKED IN STALL 406 AGAIN BUT IN A DIFFERENT PARKING LOT. THE ONE NAMED AFTER THE FORMER RED SOX OWNER TOM YAWKEY'S FAMILY. 406 WAS THE 1945 AVERAGE OF THE RED SOX'S GREAT TED WILLIAMS.

WHEN I WAS A KID TED WILLIAMS WAS THE NAME ON ALL OF THE SEARS CATALOG PICTURES OF FISHING RODS AND CAMPING TENTS.

TED WILLIAMS APPROVED ✓

I THOUGHT HE WAS A VERSION OF THE CARTOON CHARACTER MARK TRAIL.

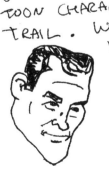

WHEN I FINALLY SAW TED'S NAME IN A LITTLE BOOK OF ALL-TIME BASEBALL GREATS I WAS SHOCKED. HOW COULD A FAT OLD FISHERMAN ALSO BE A ~~YANKEE~~ HALL OF FAME BASEBALL PLAYER? IT WAS A MOMENT OF PROFOUND PSYCHIC DISRUPTION FOR ME.

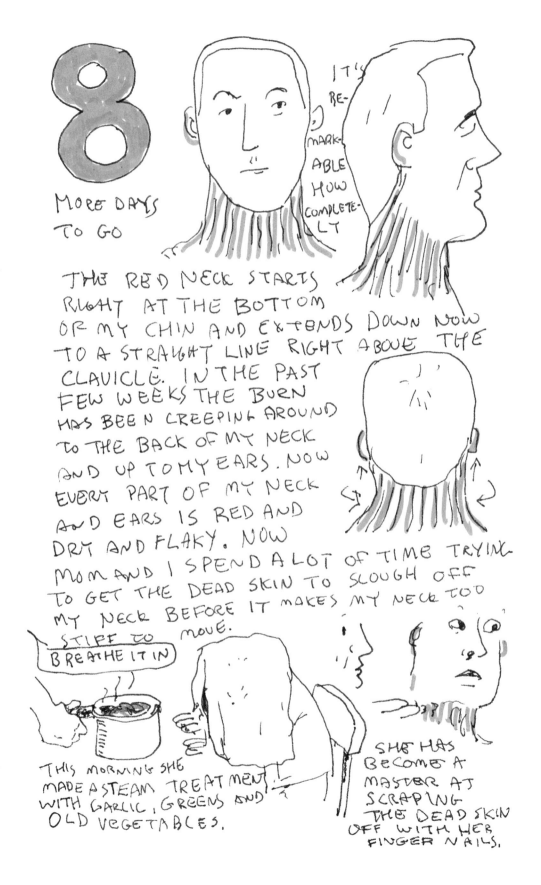

8

MORE DAYS TO GO

IT'S REMARKABLE HOW COMPLETELY

THE RED NECK STARTS RIGHT AT THE BOTTOM OF MY CHIN AND EXTENDS DOWN NOW TO A STRAIGHT LINE RIGHT ABOVE THE CLAVICLE. IN THE PAST FEW WEEKS THE BURN HAS BEEN CREEPING AROUND TO THE BACK OF MY NECK AND UP TO MY EARS. NOW EVERY PART OF MY NECK AND EARS IS RED AND DRY AND FLAKY. NOW MOM AND I SPEND A LOT OF TIME TRYING TO GET THE DEAD SKIN TO SLOUGH OFF MY NECK BEFORE IT MAKES MY NECK TOO STIFF TO MOVE.

BREATHE IT IN

THIS MORNING SHE MADE A STEAM TREATMENT WITH GARLIC, GREENS AND OLD VEGETABLES.

SHE HAS BECOME A MASTER AT SCRAPING THE DEAD SKIN OFF WITH HER FINGER NAILS.

I HAVE A FACE THAT PEOPLE CONNECT TO OTHER FACES. THE FIRST CELEBRITY I WAS COMPARED TO WAS BABY HUEY.

I WAS A FAT KID FOR A FEW YEARS. "HUSKY" IS WHAT THE SEARS CATALOG CALLED IT.

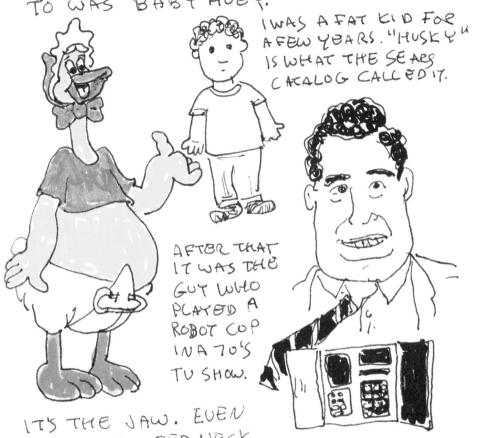

AFTER THAT IT WAS THE GUY WHO PLAYED A ROBOT COP IN A 70'S TV SHOW.

IT'S THE JAW. EVEN BEFORE MY RED NECK. I WAS CALLED HELLBOY. IT'S THE JAW.

IT'S THE RON PERLMAN

ONCE I GOT CALLED CLAIBORNE PELL, A SENATOR FROM RHODE ISLAND... IT'S THE WHITE HAIR.

THAT ACCOUNTS FOR ANDERSON COOPER AS WELL I GUESS.

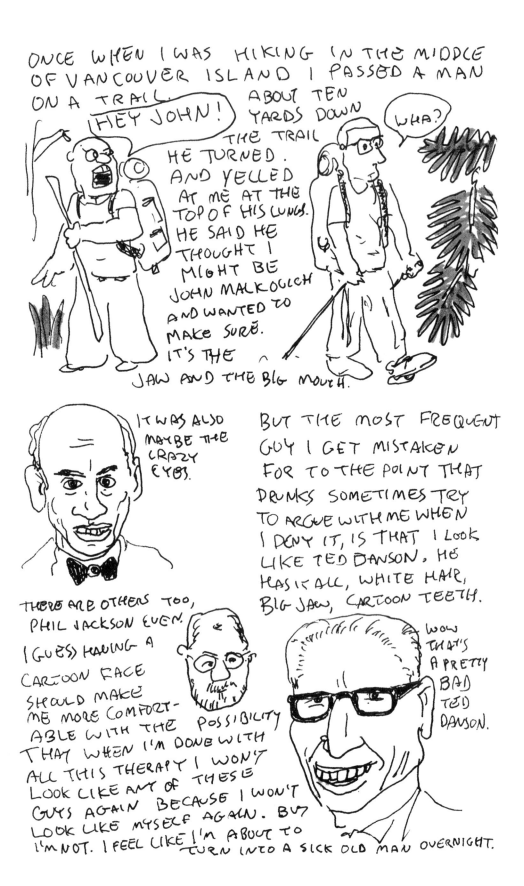

ONCE WHEN I WAS HIKING IN THE MIDDLE OF VANCOUVER ISLAND I PASSED A MAN ON A TRAIL. ABOUT TEN YARDS DOWN THE TRAIL HE TURNED. AND YELLED AT ME AT THE TOP OF HIS LUNGS. HE SAID HE THOUGHT I MIGHT BE JOHN MALKOVICH AND WANTED TO MAKE SURE. IT'S THE JAW AND THE BIG MOUTH.

HEY JOHN!

WHA?

IT WAS ALSO MAYBE THE CRAZY EYES.

THERE ARE OTHERS TOO, PHIL JACKSON EVEN. I GUESS HAVING A CARTOON FACE SHOULD MAKE ME MORE COMFORTABLE WITH THE POSSIBILITY THAT WHEN I'M DONE WITH ALL THIS THERAPY I WON'T LOOK LIKE ANY OF THESE GUYS AGAIN BECAUSE I WON'T LOOK LIKE MYSELF AGAIN. BUT I'M NOT. I FEEL LIKE I'M ABOUT TO TURN INTO A SICK OLD MAN OVERNIGHT.

BUT THE MOST FREQUENT GUY I GET MISTAKEN FOR TO THE POINT THAT DRUNKS SOMETIMES TRY TO ARGUE WITH ME WHEN I DENY IT, IS THAT I LOOK LIKE TED DANSON. HE HAS IT ALL, WHITE HAIR, BIG JAW, CARTOON TEETH.

WOW THAT'S A PRETTY BAD TED DANSON.

DAY 28   NO QUESTION | NOV 16
THIS IS THE WORST |

DAY YET. WHATEVER I WAS THINKING ON ALL THE OTHER DAYS WHEN I THOUGHT I HAD FINALLY FALLEN OFF THE CLIFF, I WAS WRONG. THIS IS WORSE. AND NOW I CAN'T IMAGINE WHAT COULD BE WORSE THAN THIS, BUT I KNOW THAT IF IT DOES, I'M DONE FOR. IT'S NOT JUST THE PAIN INSIDE BUT OUTSIDE TOO. AND THE PHLEGM IS THICKER AND STICKIER THAN EVER. I CAN'T GET IT OFF OF THE ROOF OF MY MOUTH OR OUT OF THE BACK OF MY THROAT. I THINK I MIGHT HAVE MISMANAGED MY PAIN MEDICATION BUT I CAN'T FIGURE OUT HOW. I UPPED THE ROXICET TO 12 TABLESPOONS YESTERDAY, THE MAXIMUM, I TOOK MORE DOXEPIN MOUTHWASH, WHICH BASICALLY KNOCKED ME OUT, AND I'M NOW GOING THROUGH ALMOST A BOTTLE OF MAGIC MOUTHWASH IN A DAY, BUT I CAN'T GET AHEAD OF THE PAIN NOW. I HAVEN'T UPPED THE PATCH YET, I THOUGHT I WAS SUPPOSED TO DO THAT TONIGHT, BY 50% BUT MAYBE I WAS WRONG. IN ANY CASE I'M REALLY WORRIED ABOUT GETTING THROUGH THE RADIATION SESSION TODAY, NOT TO MENTION THE FOUR THAT COME AFTER. JUST ONE DAY OFF THIS WEEK. ON SATURDAY I HAVE MY OWN VERSION OF AN ADDICTION PROBLEM NOW: I'VE

ALREADY POURED OUT MY NEXT DOSE OF ROXICET, WHICH WILL BE MY THIRD DOSE SINCE FOUR AM THIS MORNING, BUT I BETTER WAIT. IT'S ONLY ELEVEN AM AND THAT WOULD REPRESENT HALF MY ALLOWANCE FOR THE DAY. I'M ALSO LOOKING FORWARD TO TAKING THE

7

MORE DAYS TO GO

ATIVAN FOR THE RADIATION- I NEED TO RELAX, BUT SHOULD WAIT TWO MORE HOURS FOR THAT...

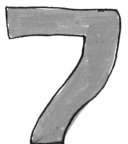

IT WAS A STRANGE DAY. BY FAR THE WORST YET, BUT I'M GETTING SO CLOSE IT'S HARD NOT TO FEEL I'M GOING TO GET THERE. MY WEIGHT WAS STILL UP, I SUFFERED THROUGH THE RADIATION, MY THROAT IS SWELLING NOW AND THE BITE BLOCK IS STARTING TO GET TIGHT) PAIN MANAGEMENT WAS OFF, BUT I THINK WE HAVE IT UNDER CONTROL TONIGHT.

LESS AIR SPACE THAN EVER

BUT NOW I'M ALMOST COMPLETELY
DRUG CONTROLLED. ALL MY WILL CAN
CONTROL IS EATING AND SCHEDULING,
I CAN'T TALK ANYMORE.
I SIT IN THE CAR LISTENING
TO MY MOTHER AND JUDY TALK.
I HAVE TO DECIDE WHAT'S WORTH
USING MY VOICE UP FOR. TURNS OUT
THERE ISN'T THAT MUCH I HAVE
TO SAY THAT IS WORTH THE PAIN
IT WILL COST ME.
   I'VE NOTICED THAT WHILE I HAVE
NO SENSE OF TASTE, I RETAIN THE
DESIRE TO LOOK AT FOOD AND
THINK ABOUT IT.
EVEN DRINKING A
BOTTLE OF ENSURE
HAS THE FAINT DISTANT BIG BANG
WHIFF OF A SENSUAL EXPERIENCE
          I DON'T FEEL HUNGER, BUT
          I CAN FEEL MYSELF FILLING
      UP, THAT'S THE CLOSEST I CAN COME
TO WHAT MIGHT BE CALLED NORMAL
DESIRE FOR FOOD.

WHAT DRIVES ME NUTS STILL IS
THE COMPLETELY NATURAL TENDENCY
PEOPLE HAVE TO GIVE ME SOMETHING
GOOD TO EAT. NOTHING IS GOOD TO
EAT. I CANNOT CHOOSE BETWEEN
COTTAGE CHEESE AND YOGURT. I DO
NOT CARE IF THERE IS A CARROT IN MY
SOUP. ADDING ICE CREAM TO AN
ENSURE SHAKE JUST MAKES IT TOO COLD
                    TO DRINK.

IT'S REMARKABLE WHAT A TRIVIAL LITTLE PERSON IS REVEALED WHEN EVERYTHING IS STRIPPED AWAY BY DRUGS AND PAIN AND FEAR. I REMEMBER BASEBALL STATISTICS AND FAMILY STORIES. I PARSE THE MEANING OF PHLEGM. THERE ISN'T A LOT OF DEEP THINKING LEFT IN ME NOW. JUST A FERAL MONKEY TRYING TO MAKE IT OUT OF THE JUNGLE. NOTHING I CAN DRINK OR SWIRL OR SPIT OUT NOW CAN FREEZE THE PAIN IN MY TONGUE. I AM WORRIED THAT WHEN I WAKE UP TOMORROW MORNING I WON'T BE ABLE

TO SWALLOW A GLASS OF WATER AND THEN I WILL BE FINISHED.

THINGS HAVE FALLEN APART. ALL I HAVE LEFT IN MY HEAD IS LITERALLY THE PAIN IN MY TONGUE. I WANT TO GET A BIGGER PICTURE, MORE PERSPECTIVE, BUT I CANNOT. ALL I CAN DO IS DWELL ON THE PAIN AND THE LIMITATIONS THE DRUGS IN MY SYSTEM HAVE PLACED ON MY IMAGINATION AND MY ABILITY TO REASON. I'M PRETTY MUCH SHOT.

I'M HOPING YESTERDAY WAS JUST A REALLY BAD DAY. AND THAT THINGS ARE BACK TO NORMAL OR WHATEVER NORMAL IS NOW. I DO HAVE TO PAY EVEN CLOSER ATTENTION THAN EVER NOW TO MY FOOD INTAKE, MY PAIN LEVELS AND MY SWALLOWING CAPACITIES IF I AM GOING TO MAKE IT THROUGH TO THE END OF THE TREATMENT SCHEDULE WITHOUT A TUBE, OR MORE IMPORTANTLY, WITHOUT INTERRUPTING THE RADIATION TREATMENTS.

TURNS OUT IT WASN'T A CLIFF. IT WAS AN ABYSS. AND I'M NOT FALLING, I'M ON A TIGHTROPE.

THE SIZE OF THE SPACE IN THE BACK OF MY THROAT THAT I CAN PASS NOURISHMENT THROUGH SEEMS TO BE SHRINKING EVERY DAY, AND MY CONTROL OVER THE BACK OF MY TONGUE, THE MUSCLE THAT IS PUSHING THE FOOD DOWN MY THROAT, IS DIMINISHING. IT ALL SEEMS TO BE PROCEEDING IN A LINEAR FASHION, LEAVING ME TO WONDER IF THE INEVITABLE RESULT IS THAT I REALLY WILL WAKE UP ONE MORNING AND FIND THAT I HAVE LOST THE ABILITY TO SWALLOW ANY FOOD. THEN I'M SUNK.

BEGINNING   MIDDLE   END?

FOOD HOLE →

TONGUE

I'M GOING NOW FOR NOT JUST A NUMBER BASED DIET, BUT AN OUTCOME BASED ONE. GETTING THROUGH THIS IS GOING TO TAKE SOME CALCULATIONS.

ASSUMPTION 1: I WANT 4000 CALORIES A DAY. I SEEM TO NEED THAT MUCH JUST TO STAY IN ONE PLACE.

ACTION I: BREAK 4000 CALORIES INTO 3 OR 4 FEEDINGS. I WAS GOING FOR 4, BUT THIS MORNING GOT 1300 CALORIES IN ONE DRINK.

THE LESS I DRINK PER CALORIE, THE EASIER IT IS TO GET DOWN THE minimum nutrition. SO THE CURRENT FORMULA:

ONE ENSURE + ONE BENECAL + DRIED GOAT MILK + 3 TBS SAFFLOWER OIL + HALF CUP WHOLE MILK

CALORIES 350 + 330 + 70 + 360 + 45 = 1155

HMM. THAT'S A LITTLE LESS THAN I THOUGHT. I MAY HAVE TO GO BACK TO THE FOUR FEEDINGS A DAY PLAN.

I'M AFRAID I'VE DEVELOPED A TOLERENCE FOR THE MAGIC MOUTHWASH. IT DOESN'T DO ITS THING ANYMORE, AND NOW I'VE STOCKPILED GALLONS OF THE STUFF.

MOM IS EATING BEET GREENS. SHE IS A HEALTHY EATER. WHAT A CONCEPT.

IF THAT STAYS AS IS, I'M IN BIG TROUBLE. IT'S HARD ENOUGH TO GET THE ENSURE DOWN NOW. WITH PAIN IT WILL BECOME IMPOSSIBLE.

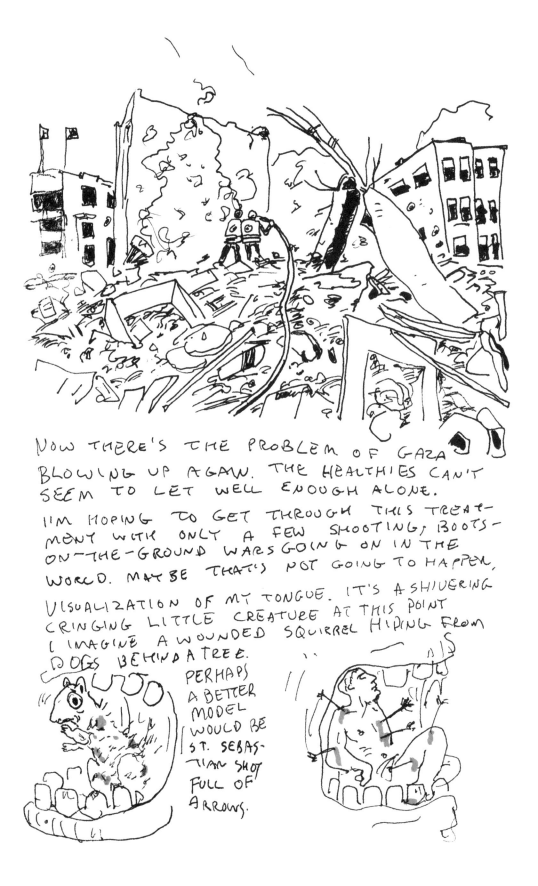

NOW THERE'S THE PROBLEM OF GAZA BLOWING UP AGAIN. THE HEALTHIES CAN'T SEEM TO LET WELL ENOUGH ALONE.

I'M HOPING TO GET THROUGH THIS TREATMENT WITH ONLY A FEW SHOOTING, BOOTS-ON-THE-GROUND WARS GOING ON IN THE WORLD. MAYBE THAT'S NOT GOING TO HAPPEN.

VISUALIZATION OF MY TONGUE. IT'S A SHIVERING CRINGING LITTLE CREATURE AT THIS POINT I IMAGINE A WOUNDED SQUIRREL HIDING FROM DOGS BEHIND A TREE.

PERHAPS A BETTER MODEL WOULD BE ST. SEBASTIAN SHOT FULL OF ARROWS.

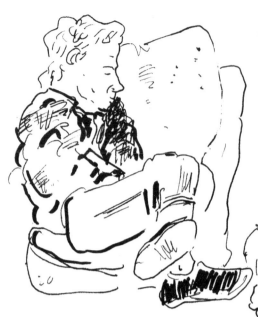

MOM CURLED UP LIKE A TEENAGER. WITH HER KINDLE. AMAZING WHAT SHE IS DOING AT 86. I'M BACK TO BEING A BABY AND SHE SEEMS TO HAVE UNLIMITED STAMINA AND ENERGY. SHE DOES LIKE TO EAT STEAK. MAYBE ALL MY THEORIES ABOUT THE ROAD TO HEALTH WERE WRONG. SHE LIKES HER STEAK RARE.

TOMORROW MORNING, SUNDAY, I'M GOING IN FOR AN EXTRA DAY OF RADIATION BECAUSE OF THE SHORT THANKSGIVING WEEK. DR. LIEBSCH GAVE ME THE OPTION OF SKIPPING THERAPY TOMORROW AND ADDING THE DAY AT THE END OF THE SCHEDULE, FINISHING ON THE 29TH INSTEAD OF THE 28TH. HE CERTAINLY SEEMED TO SUGGEST THAT WAS THE SENSIBLE THING TO DO. OTHERS CLEARLY AGREED. BUT THERE WAS NO WAY I WAS GOING TO BE ABLE TO SWITCH. I'M TERRIBLE ABOUT CHANGING PLANS IN THE MIDDLE OF A COMMITMENT AND I'M EVEN WORSE WHEN IT COMES TO BACKING OFF WHAT SEEMS LIKE A MACHO CHALLENGE. I'M NOT PROUD OF THIS. ITS A HUGE CHARACTER FLAW. I SHOULD BE MORE FLEXIBLE AND ADAPTIVE, BUT I'M NOT. I LACK THE IMAGINATION AND THE SELF CONFIDENCE TO CHANGE MY MIND. I ONLY RUN ONE WAY, AND DOWN HILL. IT GOES WITHOUT SAYING A MORE FLEXIBLE THINKER MIGHT HAVE BEEN DIAGNOSED EARLIER.

DAY 29

FIRST AND ONLY SUNDAY | NOV 18

I'M SO NERVOUS ABOUT ROLLING THE DICE ON THIS SESSION. I WOKE UP AT 1 AM, 4 AM 6 AM, 6:15 AM.

SESSION. I WENT TO BED EARLY WITH STANFORD LOSING TO THE #1 TEAM IN THE COUNTRY. NATURALLY STANFORD WON. SO SUPERSTITION, FEAR, A STAB AT MATURITY ALL COMBINED ONCE AGAIN TO ROB ME OF A PLEASANT EXPERIENCE.

I DID EMAIL MY FRIEND CATHY BEFORE GOING TO BED AND SHE STAYED UP AND WATCHED STANFORD WIN. SO AS SHE SAYS, BETWEEN US WE WERE ONE NORMAL PERSON WATCHING AND ENJOYING THE ENTIRE GAME.

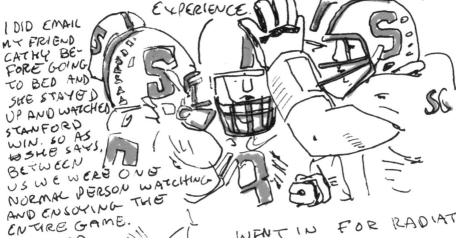

WENT IN FOR RADIATION. IT WENT BETTER THAN I EXPECTED. I THOUGHT THIS MIGHT BE A FATAL ROLL OF THE DICE, BUT INSTEAD IT WAS AN ORDINARY DAY IN ALL RESPECTS (UNLESS I'VE OVER EXTENDED MYSELF AND WILL COLLAPSE IN THE NEXT THREE DAYS).

I EVEN SEEM TO BE GETTING SOMETHING LIKE AN APPETITE BACK. I DIDN'T NOTICE AT FIRST, BUT YESTERDAY I HAD TWO BOWLS OF BROTH, THEN TODAY I HAD A LITTLE TEA, THEN SOME MUSHROOM SOUP, THEN A CUP OF YOGURT. I EVEN WENT OUT AND BOUGHT SOME CLEAR PEACH ENSURE.

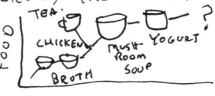

FOOD — TEA, CHICKEN BROTH, MUSHROOM SOUP, YOGURT, ?

APPETITE

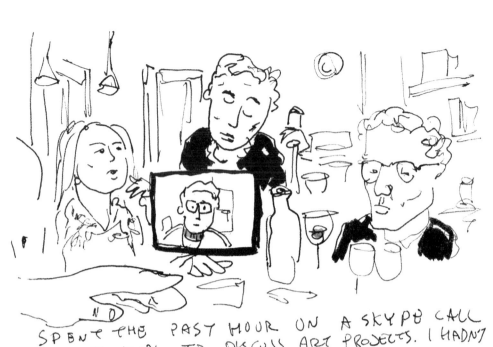

SPENT THE PAST HOUR ON A SKYPE CALL WITH FRIENDS TO DISCUSS ART PROJECTS. I HADN'T MUCH TO CONTRIBUTE, AS THOUGH I WAS A VISITOR FROM ANOTHER PLANET. IT IS GOOD THOUGH TO BEGIN TO REIMMERSE MYSELF IN THE WORLD I LEFT. AS THINGS START TO WIND DOWN ONCE AGAIN MY LIFE HOW MUCH IT'S SUDDENLY

KNOCK ON WOOD

I REALIZE HOW SIMPLE IS HERE AND MORE DIFFICULT GOING TO BE

ONCE I LEAVE. I EAT. I DRINK. I GUESS I DON'T EAT. I BRUSH MY TEETH. I GARGLE. I FLOSS. I TAKE PILLS. I PEE. I POOP. I NAP. PEOPLE WORRY ABOUT ME. THEY FEED ME, CLEAN UP AFTER ME. DRIVE ME PLACES. FORGIVE ME MY BAD MOODS. THEY TELL ME I'M DOING GREAT WHEN I'M NOT DOING ANY THING EXTRA ORDINARY. THERE IS NO TALK OF CANCER OR DEATH, EVEN, ONLY THE PROCESS COUNTS. TOO MUCH PHLEGM, NOT ENOUGH DRUGS, NOT ENOUGH CALORIES. TOO MUCH GUNK ON MY NECK. IT'S A PRETTY SWEET DEAL.

BUT JUST WHEN I GET COMPLACENT I GO ON A HACKING FIT AND ALMOST SPIT OUT MY TONGUE. I HAVE TO REMEMBER I'M STILL ON A TIGHTROPE. I FORGOT TO TAKE MY PAIN PILLS ALL DAY. I HAVE TO KEEP MY EYES DOWN FOR THE REST OF THE MONTH.

THIS MORNING IN THE PAPER THERE WAS A PIECE ABOUT PHILIP ROTH'S DECISION TO RETIRE FROM WRITING FICTION. IT'S ONE OF THE FEW THINGS I'VE READ IN THE PAST FEW MONTHS THAT BROUGHT ME UP SHORT. WHY STOP? WHY NOT DIE FIRST? HIS REASONS SEEM REASONABLE "I KNEW I WASN'T GOING TO GET AN- OTHER GOOD IDEA, OR IF I DID, I'D HAVE TO SLAVE OVER IT." ROTH'S PICTURE THAT RUNS WITH THE PIECE IS PRETTY INTER- ESTING. HE'S ALMOST 80, BUT HE'S STILL A DANDY WITH HIS DARK GELLED HAIR AND HIS NEAT LITTLE SHIRT AND SWEATER COMBO, HIS GRAY SOCKS AND HIS KHAKIS. HE'S IN CHARGE OF EVERY- THING, EVEN THE POST-IT NOTE ON HIS SCREEN IS IN CHARGE.

HOW CAN ANYONE BE SO COOL?

THE STRUGGLE WITH WRITING IS OVER.

I WILL NEVER BE SO COOL.

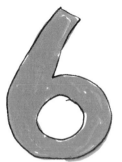

6

MORE DAYS
LEFT

AS THE BURNS GET WORSE ON THE SIDE OF MY NECK IT GETS HARDER TO DO SIMPLE THINGS. DRIVING IS HARD BECAUSE I CAN'T TWIST MY NECK.

THERE IS NO HAIR THERE AND ITS

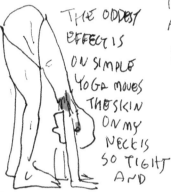

THE ODDEST EFFECT IS ON SIMPLE YOGA MOVES THE SKIN ON MY NECK IS SO TIGHT AND PAINFUL I CAN'T FULLY EXTEND MY ARMS FULLY UP OR OR DOWN

AS DRY AS A DESERT. EVERY WRINKLE BECOMES A CREASE, EVERY CREASE BECOMES A FOLD AND EVERY FOLD FEELS LIKE A PAPER CUT

WHEN I START TO GAG THOUGH, IS WHEN IT GETS SCARY. RETCHING OR GAGGING REQUIRE THE MUSCLES IN THE NECK TO SPASM BUT WHEN THAT HAPPENS TO ME IT FEELS LIKE MY HEAD IS GOING TO FLY OFF BEFORE I CAN GET THE BLOB OF MUCUS UP AND OUT OF MY THROAT. THAT'S WHAT SCARES ME - THAT ALL THAT WILL HAPPEN WHILE I HAVE THE MASK ON AND I'M BEING RADIATED THERE WOULD BE AT LEAST THREE POSSIBLE HORRIBLE DEATHS

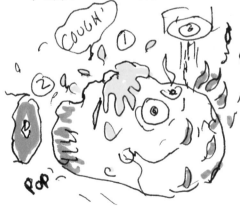

IN THAT SCENARIO.
1. DROWNING BY PHLEGM
2. HEAD FALLS OFF
3. BURNT TO DEATH BY MISPLACED PROTON BEAM

DAY 30 A DEFINITE WATERSHED DAY

30 OUT OF 35 $\frac{6}{7}$ OF THE WAY THROUGH

EARLIEST DAY OF RADIATION YET: 8:20 AM
UP AT 4:15 SPITTING AND HACKING.
THE NEXT THREE DAYS ARE MY FOCUS NOW:
4000 CALORIES A DAY, LOTS OF DRUGS FOR THE
RADIATION.

I BEGAN RETCHING
IN THE MORNING
AND FOR A MOMENT
I THOUGHT I WOULD
EITHER BUST A
BLOOD VESSEL IN
MY NECK OR
THROW UP MY 1045
CALORIE MORNING
DRINK

BUT I GOT THROUGH IT.
I NOW HAVE AS ELABORATE A PRE RADIATION
ROUTINE AS A BASEBALL PLAYER STEPPING
UP TO THE PLATE. THE IDEA IS THE SAME
IN MANY WAYS: TO FOCUS AND TAKE
THE PERSONAL OUT OF THE PROCESS. OF
COURSE IN MY CASE DRUGS DON'T HURT!
70 MINUTES BEFORE RADIATION
POP THE PILL. ABOUT 40
MINUTES LATER I START TO
FEEL LIKE I'M IN A WARM BATH
30 MINUTES BEFORE RADIATION AT PROTON
CENTER. GARGLE THEN,
BRUSH
TEETH
FLOSS TEETH
2 TBS ROXICET
SPRITZ UP EACH NOSTRIL
WITH NASAL SPRAY
MORE BRUSHING.
THEN. 1 MINUTE BEFORE
A LAST GARGLE WITH MAGIC MOUTHWASH
AND ANOTHER ATTEMPT TO HAWK UP PHLEGM

HAUWKK!

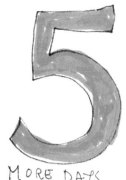

5

MORE DAYS
LEFT

LET'S FACE IT. THESE FOUR PAGES A DAY HAVE BECOME AS MUCH OF A SUSTAINING DISTRACTING ROUTINE AS MY RADIATION SHENANIGANS OR MY CALORIE COUNTING FOOD INTAKE SYSTEM. WHEN I BEGAN I THOUGHT I WOULD MEANDER FROM ONE TOPIC TO ANOTHER AND PRODUCE A BUNCH OF PAGES ALMOST WITHOUT NOTICING. BY THE THIRD DAY OF TREATMENT THOUGH I COULD TELL THAT THE TAIL WOULD WAG THE DOG: TRYING TO FILL THE NOTEBOOK EVERY DAY WOULD BECOME AS MUCH OF A ROUTINE, AND ANXIETY AND SATISFACTION, AS ANY OF MY OTHER

ROUTINES
WRITING
SMALLER

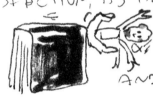

FIRST THE ITSELF GOT AND TIGHTER. I BECAME MORE RESISTANT TO LEAVING OPEN SPACES ON THE PAGE. I BECAME LESS ENCHANTED WITH QUICK ~~drawn~~ SLOPPY CARTOONY DRAWINGS AND 'DRAWN' TO MORE TIGHTLY PRESENTED PICTURES. I ALSO FOUND THAT AS THE DIFFICULTY OF THE TREATMENT RAMPED UP AND I HAD TO RESPOND BY CHANGING MY DIET AND MY SLEEPING HABITS AND MY TOLERANCE FOR PAIN MEDICATION, THAT I COULD NO LONGER SUSTAIN LONG COMPLICATED THOUGHTS OR ARGUMENTS OR EVEN SENTENCES. I HAD TO MOVE REACTIVELY FROM ONE THING TO THE NEXT.

I HOPE IN THE MORNING THAT SOMETHING INTERESTING HAPPENS THAT I CAN DRAW WHILE I AM STILL ALERT. THAT MAY ACCOUNT FOR THE DISPROPORTIONATE APPEARANCE OF BASEBALL PLAYERS AND BASEBALL STATISTICS RELATED TO THE MORNING PARKING SITUATION

SOMETIME IN THE DAY I LOOK FORWARD TO SOME EVENT OR IMAGE THAT WILL LEND ITSELF TO AN ENTRY IN THE BOOK. BUT THESE DAYS I RARELY HAVE THE TIME OR ENERGY TO WORK ON THE BOOK BEFORE LATE NIGHT. OFTEN AT TEN PM

TODAY WE PARKED IN STALL 38

FRANK THOMAS HIT 38 HOME RUNS ONCE 1994? BUT WHO CARES?

OR SO I AM LEFT LOOKING AT ONE ☐ TWO. ☐☐, OR THREE ☐☐☐ BLANK SHEETS. AND I'M TIRED AND SORE AND DISCOURAGED. NOT A GOOD COMBINATION FOR A MEMOIRIST.

THE POINT NOW THOUGH IS NO LONGER TO DISCOVER OR RELATE SOME INSIGHT INTO MY DISEASE OR MY LIFE, THE POINT NOW IS SIMPLY TO DRAW IN THE BOOK ITSELF. THE BOOK IS HELPING ME GET THROUGH THIS. IT'S ANOTHER ARBITRARY OBSESSION I CAN FOCUS ON

TO KEEP ME FROM THINKING ABOUT
BIGGER AND MORE DIFFICULT THINGS.

I DID GET GOOD NEWS TODAY.

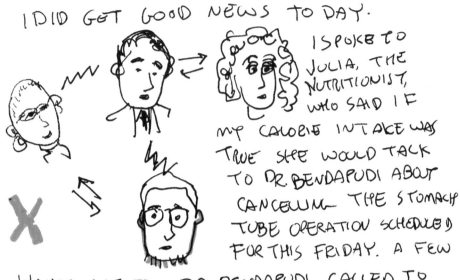

I SPOKE TO
JULIA, THE
NUTRITIONIST,
WHO SAID IF
MY CALORIE INTAKE WAS
TRUE SHE WOULD TALK
TO DR. BENDAPUDI ABOUT
CANCELLING THE STOMACH
TUBE OPERATION SCHEDULED
FOR THIS FRIDAY. A FEW
HOURS LATER DR. BENDAPUDI CALLED TO
SAY HE WOULD RECOMMEND TO DR. WIRTH
THAT WE CANCEL THE OPERATION.

SO THAT'S IT. THAT'S THE BIG THING
I'VE BEEN FIGHTING TO ACHIEVE FOR THE
PAST FIVE WEEKS. I HAVE SUCCEEDED. I SHOULD
BE HAPPY, BUT NATURALLY I'M NOT. I'M
WORRIED NOW BECAUSE OF BEING ABLE TO
COMPETE AGAINST THEIR EXPECTATIONS I
NOW HAVE TO LIVE UP TO THEM. IF I
FAIL NOW I LET EVERYONE DOWN, NOT JUST
MYSELF. I'LL GIVE MYSELF A BIT OF A
BREAK HERE AND NOT CHALK THIS UP TO
MY NORMAL SELF-DEFEATING PESSIMISM.
I'M IN THE BOTTOM OF THE MONDAY
NIGHT DIP. PAIN IS AT ITS WEEKLY
HIGH POINT, SUSTAINING DRUGS AT THEIR
LOWEST. I'M GOING TO FILL MYSELF UP WITH
AS MANY PAIN MASKING DRUGS AS I CAN
LAY MY HANDS ON AND GO TO BED.

TODAY I ANTICIPATE (BAD MOVE) HAVING 31 DOWN AND 4 TO GO. THAT'S A RECORD OF 31-4 WHICH WAS LEFTY GROVE'S RECORD IN 1931. I ALWAYS THOUGHT THAT WAS A VERY ELEGANT RECORD. AN OUTRAGEOUS NUMBER OF WINS AND A MINISCULE NUMBER OF LOSSES

(31-4)

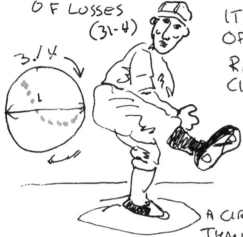

3.14

IT'S ALSO THE BEGINNING OF PI 3.14, THE RATIO OF A CIRCLE'S CIRCUMFERENCE TO ITS DIAMETER

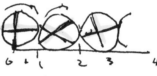

0 1 2 3 4

A CIRCLE IS A LITTLE MORE THAN THREE TIMES LONGER AROUND THAN IT IS ACROSS.

THESE DAYS PI IS ALSO LIFE OF PI, THE NOVEL

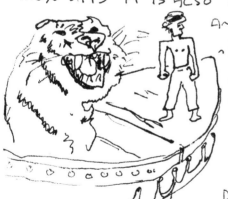

AND MOVIE ABOUT A MAN STUCK ON A LIFEBOAT WITH A BENGAL TIGER — THAT'S ALSO ABOUT TRUTH AND GOD AND YADA YADA ANOTHER MOVIE / BOOK TO LOOK AT LATER, WHEN EVERYTHING SETTLES DOWN

I'M IN A SEMI PERMANENT DAZE NOW AS I STAGGER TOWARDS THE FINISH LINE. MY TONGUE AND THROAT ARE COMPLETELY RAW AND TO KEEP UP WITH THE PAIN I HAVE TO KEEP UPPING THE PATCHES.
I DON'T WANT TO, BECAUSE I DON'T WANT TO SLEEP THROUGH THE LAST WEEK OF MY THERAPY, BUT I DON'T WANT TO BE AN IDIOT AND BLOW EVERYTHING AT THE LAST MINUTE.

25 msg/HR

50 msg/HR

25 msg/HR

I MISSED SEEING AN OLD SILENT PETER PAN MOVIE LAST NIGHT BECAUSE I WASN'T FEELING VERY WELL. JUDY SENT ME A SHORT EXCERPT FROM THE MOVIE THOUGH THAT INCLUDES A SHOT OF MERMAIDS ON THE ROCKS THAT I LOVE. THERE ARE SO MANY MERMAIDS AND THEY ARE ALL JUST LYING THERE ON THE ROCKS AND THE CAMERA DOESN'T REALLY CARE WHICH ONE YOU LOOK AT, JUST THAT YOU LOOK AT THEM ALL. IT'S VERY BLURRY, BUT I THINK THAT'S PETER PAN HIMSELF IN THE VERY MIDDLE. TO ME, THIS LOOKS MORE LIKE A NATIONAL GEO-GRAPHIC PICTURE OF BASKING WALRUSES THAN ANYTHING ELSE.

THESE LAST FEW DAYS ARE LIVING UP TO THEIR PROMISE EVEN AS I GET CLOSE ENOUGH TO THE END TO BEGIN PLANNING ON MY EXIT STRATEGY. MY SYMPTOMS ARE PILING UP NOW AND I CAN'T SEE MY WAY CLEAR TO A GOOD FEW DAYS THAT WILL GET ME OVER THE HUMP.

MY TONGUE IS WORSE THAN EVER. I LEAVE IT ALONE FOR EVEN A FEW MINUTES AND IT DRIES UP, GETS COVERED IN GOO, FEELS LIKE A FOREST FIRE. THIS MORNING IT LOOKED LIKE A LITTLE MONK WITH A YELLOW CLOAK AND YELLOW GOO A BRIGHT RED FACE. MY TONGUE BARELY CAN POKE ¼ BEYOND MY TEETH WITHOUT STARTING TO QUIVER AND SHAKE AND PULL BACK

MY NECK DRIES OUT IN MINUTES TOO, UNLESS I SLATHER ON THE VASELINE LIKE AQUAPHOR IT GETS SO STIFF I CANT LOOK RIGHT OR LEFT ITS LIKE A GIANT CLAMP HAS BEEN PRESSED ONTO MY NECK

THE NECK IS SO SWOLLEN NOW THAT THE MASK IS LEAVING DEEP WAFFLE-LIKE IMPRESSIONS THAT ARE LASTING LONGER AND LONGER CHIN WAFFLES NOSE WAFFLES NECK AND CHIN WAFFLES

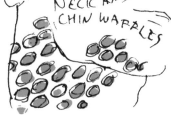

4

MORE DAYS
TO GO

I STOPPED TALKING FOR THE MOST PART. THERE ARE VERY FEW THINGS I WANT TO SAY NOW THAT ARE WORTH THE PAIN I HAVE TO ENDURE TO SAY THEM. I'LL HAVE TO REMEMBER THAT LATER WHEN I'M BACK TO NORMAL AND EAGER TO TELL EVERY-ONE WHAT I THINK ABOUT NOTHING IN PARTICULAR. THE DANGER WHEN YOU DON'T SPEAK IS THAT PEOPLE ASSUME YOU DON'T HAVE AN OPINION, OR AT LEAST NOT ONE YOU CARE ENOUGH ABOUT TO DEFEND BY TALKING. I CAN SEE WHY LITTLE OLD MEN AND WOMEN GET SO GLUM LOOKING. EVERYONE IS ALWAYS TELLING THEM WHAT THEY THINK.

TOMORROW IS A BIG, BIG DAY.

JOSH + TOM + FAMILIES FLY IN, I GO TO RADIATION AT 8:30 AM, THEN MEET AND HOPEFULLY BURY THE STOMACH TUBE WITH DRS WIRTH + BENDAPUDI FOR ONCE AND FOR ALL. THEN A LONG CHEMO SESSION. THEN A FAMILY REUNION. I HOPE I DON'T FALL APART. I CAN REALLY USE THE FOUR DAY BREAK THOUGH. I'M NOT WORKING WITH A FULL SET OF SPARK PLUGS.

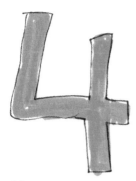

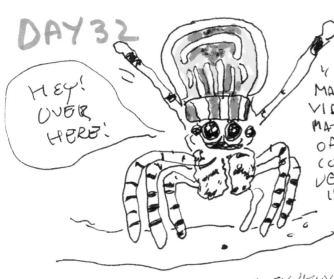

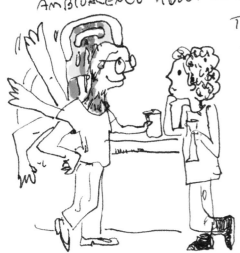

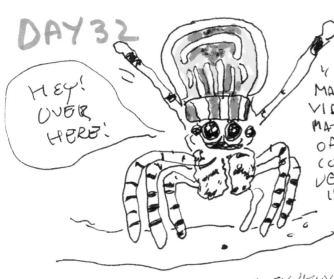

DAY 32

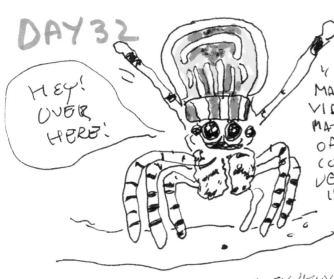

HEY! OVER HERE!

MARY SENT ME A VIDEO OF THE MATING DANCE OF THE PEA-COCK SPIDER. VERY INSPIRING. I'M SORE ALL OVER, BUT THIS IS A GOOD SIGN, GETTING INTO INSECT SEX RITUALS

WHO KNOWS WHY ANIMALS FIGHTING OR MATING GIVE US SUCH A KICK? HARD NOT TO SEE THEM AS PLUCKY LITTLE PEOPLE WHO AREN'T AFRAID TO DISPENSE WITH OUR NEUROTIC AMBIVALENCE ABOUT OUR DESIRES AND JUST GO FOR IT

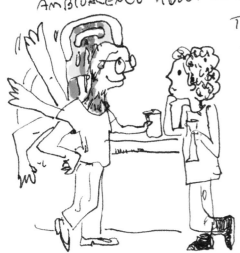

THAT'S ABOUT ALL I'VE GOT. TODAY IS THE FIRST MECHANICAL FAILURE OF THIS THERAPY. I WAS HALFWAY THROUGH THE SESSION, IN A PRETTY GOOD BUZZ, FALLING ASLEEP EVEN, WHEN THE GANTRY MACHINERY FROZE AND THEY TOOK ME OFF OF THE GURNEY AND EXILED ME BACK INTO THE WAITING ROOM. SO NOW WE JUST SIT HERE WAITING FOR THEM TO FIGURE OUT WHAT'S WRONG. I HOPE THIS DOESN'T SOMEHOW AFFECT THE BALANCE OF THE TREATMENTS AS THIS HAS PROGRESSED AND I HAVE RESPONDED BY BECOMING MORE SYSTEMATIC AND REGIMENTED IN MY PREPARATIONS AND HABITS, I HAVE TRIED NOT TO THINK ABOUT WHAT WOULD HAPPEN WHEN EVENTS OUT-SIDE MY CONTROL, STORMS, ILLNESS, MECHANICAL BREAKDOWNS INTERFERED WITH PROGRESS. TOO MANY UNKNOWNS TO KNOW.

LAST NIGHT I WATCHED THE NEW
SHERLOCK HOLMES ON THE IPAD WITH MOM.
EVEN THOUGH IT WAS A STYLISH AND WITTY
BRAIN TEASER WITH LOTS OF THINGS TO KEEP →
ME INTERESTED - EVEN APPARENTLY A GOLEM
THAT ATTACKED HOLMES AND WATSON,

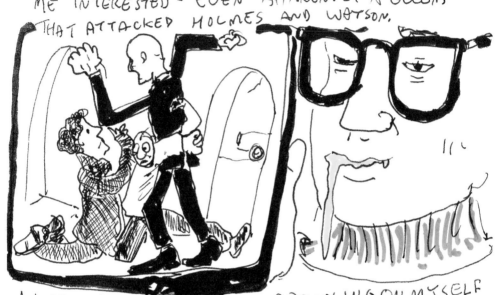

I KEPT NODDING OFF AND DROOLING ON MYSELF
I COULDN'T FOLLOW THE ACTION. MOM COULDN'T
FOLLOW EITHER BUT SHE DIDN'T DROOL ON HERSELF
SO. THEY PUT ME IN ANOTHER GANTRY
IDENTICAL TO THE FIRST EXCEPT FOR TWO
MISSING PANELS I THINK.

SPOT THE DIFFERENCE

GANTRY 1   GANTRY 2

THEN WE MET WITH
DRS WIRTH AND BENDAPUDI
AND THEY OFFICIALLY CANCELLED THE TUBE INSERTION
IN FINE FORM
JOSH AND TOM ARRIVED   THE DAY.
AND GOT ME THROUGH

SLEEPY   HAPPY

JUDE AND FLEURRY   DROVE UP AND
OUR PACK IS BACK TOGETHER. JUDE SUGGESTS
UPPING THE DRAWN-ON RING MOTIF BY
GETTING OURSELVES WEDDING RING

TATOOS. 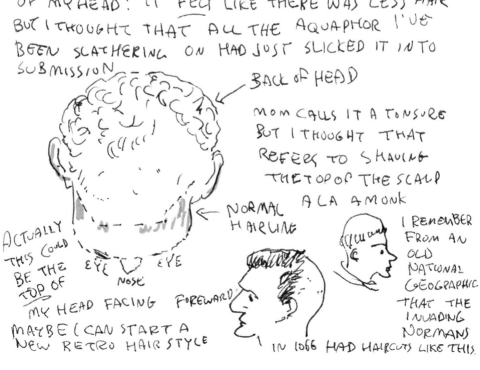 I WILL HAVE
TO THINK ON THIS. I DEF-
INITELY ONE HER ONE, HAVING
DRAGGED HER DOWN TO CITY HALL WITH ONLY
A SILVER SHARPIE PEN FOR OUR VOWS,
BUT I HATE TATOOS. SO PERMANENT AND SO
ARBITRARY. MAYBE I WILL COUNTER PROPOSE
THAT WE DO THE TATTOOS OURSELVES, PRISON
STYLE. THAT WOULD BE REALLY PERSONAL
AND WE'D BOTH LEARN A NEW SKILL.

DOUBLE LINE   TEAR DROPS   BARBED WIRE   GREEK PATTERN

WE NEED DESIGN IDEAS

JUDE ALSO DISCOVERED SOMETHING THAT
NO ONE ELSE HAS IN THE LAST FEW WEEKS:
I'VE BEEN LOSING HAIR ALONG THE BACK
OF MY HEAD! IT FELT LIKE THERE WAS LESS HAIR
BUT I THOUGHT THAT ALL THE AQUAPHOR I'VE
BEEN SLATHERING ON HAD JUST SLICKED IT INTO
SUBMISSION

BACK OF HEAD

MOM CALLS IT A TONSURE
BUT I THOUGHT THAT
REFERS TO SHAVING
THE TOP OF THE SCALP
A LA A MONK

NORMAL HAIRLINE

ACTUALLY THIS COULD
BE THE
TOP OF   EYE   EYE
NOSE
MY HEAD FACING FOREWARD

MAYBE I CAN START A
NEW RETRO HAIR STYLE

I REMEMBER
FROM AN
OLD
NATIONAL
GEOGRAPHIC
THAT THE
INVADING
NORMANS
IN 1066 HAD HAIRCUTS LIKE THIS.

3

I HOPE WE HAVEN'T RUN MOM DOWN. SHE HAS SO MUCH ENERGY AND DRIVE IT'S ALL TOO EASY TO FORGET SHE IS 86 AND ONLY A YEAR AND A HALF PAST BREAST CANCER AND A DOUBLE MASTECTOMY HERSELF. SHE HAS A COLD NOW AND SHE'S REALLY KNOCKED OUT. BUT OF COURSE SHE WON'T ALLOW PLANS TO BE CHANGED ON HER BEHALF, ONLY ON MINE AND OF COURSE I WON'T ADMIT THAT I'M TIRED EITHER WHICH FREQUENTLY GETS US IN MESSES. I WON'T GIVE IN, AND SHE WON'T SO WE OVERDO IT AND SHE CRASHES AND I WORRY THAT I'VE KILLED HER. THEN SHE POPS UP AGAIN GOOD AS NEW A COUPLE OF HOURS LATER AND I FEEL LIKE AN IDIOT. I GUESS I KNOW WHERE I GOT THIS REALITY-OVERCOMING STOICISM.

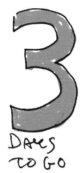

ABE BET JUDE $5 LAST MONTH WHEN THEY WERE VISITING THAT HIS ALREADY VERY LOOSE TOOTH WOULD ~~BE~~ ~~STILL~~ STILL BE HANGING IN THERE WHEN HE RETURNED FOR THANKSGIVING. HE JUST SENT HER A PICTURE TO PROVE IT'S STILL HANGING IN THERE THE DAY BEFORE THANKSGIVING. HE GOT HIT BY HIS COUSIN THOUGH AND IT'S BARELY THERE. WE COULD SLIP THE COUSIN A COUPLE OF BUCKS TO MAKE IT GO AWAY PERMANENTLY HE WAS IN TEARS, ABE, WAS. "WHY DO BABY TEETH HAVE TO DIE?" FOR ME, BABY TEETH WERE THE LAST DO-OVER, THE LAST TIME I THOUGHT THE UNIVERSE WAS LOOKING OUT FOR ME. WRECK ALL YOUR TEETH AS A BABY? NO PROBLEM. YOU GET TO START ALL OVER AGAIN WITH A BRAND NEW SET. IMMORTALITY.

THIS IS A DATE THAT IS ITS OWN MNEMONIC DEVICE: EVERY YEAR | NOV 22

WE COUNT BACK TO WHERE WE WERE. I WAS IN FIRST GRADE AND THE TEACHER SHOWED US THE SCHOOL FLAG WAS AT HALF MAST. "BECAUSE THE PRESIDENT HAS BEEN SHOT."

I THOUGHT SHE MEANT THE PRINCIPAL OF THE SCHOOL HAD BEEN SHOT. I COULD NOT IMAGINE THAT THE WORLD OF SCHOOL, THE KID WORLD, AND THE WORLD OF ADULTS WOULD EVER OVERLAP

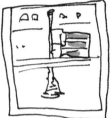

NEXT YEAR WILL BE HALF A CENTURY SINCE.

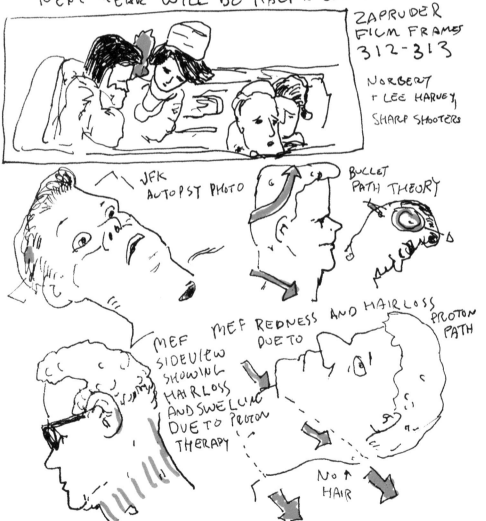

ZAPRUDER FILM FRAMES 312-313

NORBERT + LEE HARVEY, SHARP SHOOTERS

JFK AUTOPSY PHOTO

BULLET PATH THEORY

MEF MEF REDNESS AND HAIRLOSS DUE TO SIDEVIEW SHOWING HAIRLOSS AND SWELLING DUE TO PROTON THERAPY

PROTON PATH

NOT HAIR

WHEN I WAS KID I WOULD BRING MY LITTLE
CLAY FIGURES HOME FROM ART CLASS TO
SHOW MY PARENTS. THEY NEVER DISAPPOINTED
ME – OOHING AND AAHING OVER EACH AND
EVERY PIECE.

IT'S CALLED "WOE"

IT'S VERY SAD

BUT ITS ALSO BEAUTIFUL MATTY

I GOT USED TO HAVING THEM TELL ME HOW WONDER-
FUL EVERYTHING I MADE WAS. BY THE TIME I LEFT
FOR COLLEGE MY PARENTS HAD BUILT EXTRA SHELVES
TO HOLD ALL THE FIGURES. MOST OF THEM WERE SEMI
NUDE MALE FIGURES
INSPIRED BY MY ADMIRATION
FOR CLASSICAL GREEK POTTERY +
DONATELLO SCULPTURE – I
THINK MICHAELANGELO
AND RODIN WERE ALWAYS
TOO RICH FOR MY BLOOD

ZUCCONE
PUMPKIN
HEAD

FREEDMAN

AS I STUDIED ART IN SCHOOLS
AND BECAME MORE AWARE
OF THE PLACE MY WORK
HAD IN CRAFT AND OUT-
SIDER TRADITIONS, THE
LESS COMFORTABLE I BE-
CAME WITH MY SENTIMENTAL
ROOTS IN A KIND OF HALF-
BAKED ROMANTICISM. BUT

BUST

STILL I'VE NEVER BEEN ABLE TO SHAKE COMPLETELY
THE FIGURE OUT OF MY WORK OR THE STORY TELLING
QUALITY, OR THE APPEAL TO SENTIMENTAL AND
ROMANTIC IDEAS ABOUT ART. IT MARKS ME
AS AN ECCENTRIC AND KIND OR BOXES ME
IN AS A CONTEMPORARY ARTIST.

THE OTHER THING I'M LEFT WITH IS THE ANXIETY OVER EVERY PIECE I MAKE. I FEEL I'M STILL BRINGING EVERYTHING HOME FOR APPROVAL. ITS THE WORST WAY TO MAKE ART, ALWAYS TRYING TO MAKE SOMETHING GOOD. YOU CAN'T EXPERIMENT. YOU CLOSE DOWN, YOU REPEAT YOURSELF. I SEE THIS IN STUDENTS ALL THE TIME. I'M ALWAYS TRYING TO DEVISE TRICKS ("MAKE A TERRIBLE WORK OF ART!") TO FORCE THEM TO TAKE RISKS SO THEY CAN GROW BECAUSE THAT'S STILL MY OWN GREATEST PROBLEM: THAT I WANT APPROVAL FOR EVERY PIECE I MAKE.

SO I MAKE LOTS OF PIECES VERY FAST, VERY SMALL, VERY SLOPPY. I GIVE THEM AWAY. I TRY NOT TO MAKE THEM COUNT FOR MUCH. BUT STILL, MY FAMILY LOVES ME TOO MUCH NOT TO LOVE EVERYTHING I MAKE. I FINISHED THOSE NINE GIFTS TO MY CARETAKERS PLUS THREE OTHERS AND PAINTED THEM GOLD. MY MOTHER WROTE NOTES ON EACH OF THEM AND THEN ASKED ME TO RECORD A VIDEO DESCRIBING EACH ONE SO SHE COULD SHARE IT WITH OUR FRIENDS AND FAMILY. I AGREED, BUT I DON'T HAVE MUCH OF A VOICE LEFT NOW.

THIS IS A MAN STICKING HIS TONGUE OUT FOR DR. LIEBSCH.

THE FIRST TAKE WAS WITH MY MOTHER'S IPHONE WHICH DOESN'T HAVE MUCH OF A MICROPHONE SO THAT DIDN'T WORK. THEN WE DID A WHOLE TAKE WITHOUT TURNING ON THE CAMERA. FINALLY WE GOT SOMETHING DOWN. I FELT LIKE I WAS NINE YEARS OLD AGAIN

WE WENT OVER TO EDEN AND
PETER AND NATHAN AND OLLIE AND
BELLA'S FOR THANKSGIVING THIS AFTERNOON.
I BROUGHT THEM THE TINY GOLD TURKEY
I MADE. THAT WAS ABOUT
THE LAST ACTIVE GESTURE
I MADE DURING THE AFTERNOON.
MY THROAT CLOSED UP AND I SAT
THERE LIKE A LUMP. FOR THE PAST
FEW WEEKS I'VE BEEN WORRYING ABOUT
THIS AFTERNOON. I DIDN'T WANT TO
SCARE MY NIECES AND NEPHEWS BY
BEING TOO SICK OR OUT OF IT. I DIDN'T
REALLY EXPECT TO BE, BUT I THINK I
WAS. I COULDN'T TALK AT ALL. I JUST
SAT THERE WITH MY LITTLE NECK
GAITER ON TO HIDE MY BURN MARKS
I MANAGED TO DRINK FOUR
BOTTLES OF ENSURE DURING
DINNER. THAT'S 1400 CALORIES
I WONDER HOW THAT COMPARES
TO WHAT I WOULD HAVE
EATEN ON A NORMAL
THANKSGIVING. PETER
THOUGHT AN AVERAGE
PLATE
OF FOOD
WOULD
HAVE
AROUND 400
CALORIES, SO
I WAS AT LEAST IN
THE BALL PARK
PIG-OUT WISE.

ENSURE

MACARONI
AND CHEESE

STUFFED
PORTABELLO
MUSHROOM

GREEN
BEANS

THIS
EVENING
FLEURRY THREW
UP ON MY HAT AND
I KIND OF LOST IT IN
MY SQUEAKY LITTLE
DRY MOUTH VOICE
I GOTTA WATCH
IT. I'M SLIPPING.

MASHED
POTATOES

TURKEY

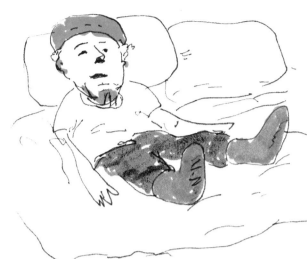

SLOW MORNING AS PEOPLE RECOVER FROM THANKSGIVING. SLEPT A LITTLE BETTER LAST

NIGHT, BUT I'VE BECOME ALMOST COMPLETELY SILENT. THERE IS A NEW CRITERIA FOR USING MY VOICE — TONGUE-WORTHINESS

NOT MUCH I HAVE TO SAY IS WORTH THE TOLL IT TAKES ON MY TONGUE.

WE ALL CONVERGED ON

NORTH BRIDGE THIS AFTERNOON TO LOOK AT THE SPOT WHERE THE AMERICAN REVOLUTION BEGAN WITH THE SHOT HEARD ROUND THE WORLD. IT'S NOT THAT MUCH TO LOOK AT, TURNS OUT. A CREAKY WOODEN BRIDGE — NOT THE ORIGINAL ONE EVEN OVER THE THIN LITTLE RIVER

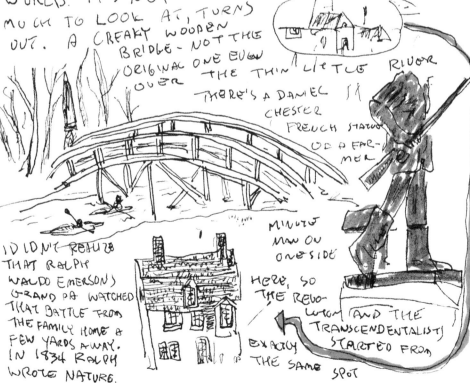

THERE'S A DANIEL CHESTER FRENCH STATUE OF A FARMER

MINUTE MAN ON ONE SIDE

HERE, SO THE REVOLUTION AND THE TRANSCENDENTALISTS STARTED FROM EXACTLY THE SAME SPOT

I DIDN'T REALIZE THAT RALPH WALDO EMERSON'S GRANDPA WATCHED THAT BATTLE FROM THE FAMILY HOME A FEW YARDS AWAY. IN 1834 RALPH WROTE NATURE.

THE NIECES AND NEPHEWS WERE LESS INTERESTED IN EITHER THE REVOLUTION OR THE BIRTH OF TRANSCENDENTALISM THAN IN WRESTLING FOR THE ATTENTION OF PEACHIE, THE SMALLEST OF THEM ALL, BUT A DOMINATING PERSONALITY ALREADY. THEY LOVED CARTING HER ALL OVER THE PARK. AS AN ICONIC PATRIOTIC ~~SITE,~~ SIGHT, IT WAS ODDLY FAMILIAR.

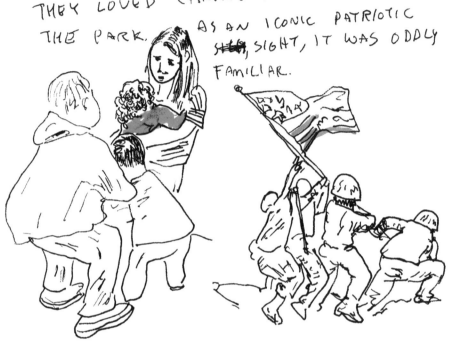

I'M ALMOST COMPLETELY DISFUNCTIONAL NOW. I CAN ONLY REALLY DO A COUPLE OF THINGS NOW. DRINK CALORIES AND BRUSH MY TEETH. EVERYTHING ELSE IS A DISTANT MEMORY. I COMMUNICATE, WHEN I BOTHER, WITH SIGN LANGUAGE. I AM LOOKING FORWARD FOR SOME REASON, TO AN ABSOLUTELY TERRIBLE MEAL AT THE END OF ALL THIS. SODA POP, A GREASY SANDWICH AND ANOTHER GREASY SANDWICH. I DON'T EVEN KNOW THE PARTICULARS. BUT THE IDEA OF ENJOYING SOMETHING SWEET AND TINGLY, AND THE NOTION THAT SOMETHING MIGHT ACTUALLY TASTE SO GOOD I'D WANT TO EAT IT TWICE IS IRRESISTABLE.

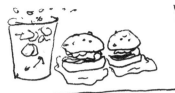

THIS EVENING JOSH AND MOM AND I DROVE OVER TO SEE THE LEAVYS AGAIN TODAY. STAN LEAVY WAS IN TOWN. STAN AND MY FATHER WERE FRIENDS AND COLLEAGUES AT YALE OVER 60 YEARS AGO. THEY WENT THROUGH PSYCHO-ANALYTIC TRAINING TOGETHER. STAN AND MARGARET'S YOUNG FAMILY HAD A GREAT IMPACT ON MY FATHER, AND MY MOTHER AND FATHER HAD A BIG IMAACT ON THE LEAVY KIDS. WE LOVED THE LEAVY KIDS WHEN WE WERE YOUNG - WE LOOKED UP TO THEM JONATHAN LEAVY SHOWED ME HOW TO OPEN A BANK ACCOUNT SHOWON AND VIVI LEAVY ME HOW TO DO MY LAUNDRY WHEN JOSH WENT TO COLLEGE STAN AND MARGARET WOULD IN- VITE HIM OVER AND SERVE HIM SHERRY. THEY MADE HIM FEEL LIKE AN ADULT. THEY WERE VERY CLOSE, BUT NOT SO MUCH AT THE END OF MY FATHER'S LIFE. HE DIED IN 2004. STAN IS STILL GOING STRONG AT 97.

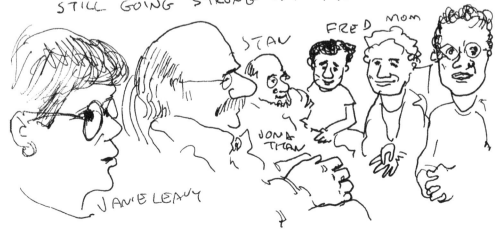

WHEN I GOT HOME JUDE WENT TO
WALGREEN'S AND CAME HOME WITH
A DVD OF THREE STOOGES SHORTS
THAT WAS PERFECT.

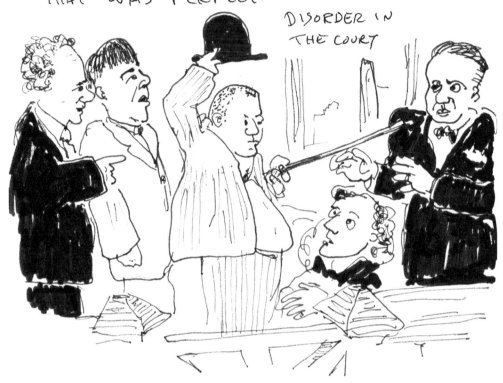

DISORDER IN
THE COURT

HALFWAY THROUGH THE LAST LONG WEEKEND
OF THE TREATMENT. I WAS HOPING FOR
A MIRACULOUS RECOUPERATION THAT WOULD
LET THE LAST THREE DAYS OF TREATMENT
FLY BY WITHOUT DRAMA. NOT SO SURE I'M
GOING TO GET THAT LAST LITTLE BREAK.
DRINKING THE ENSURE IS DRIVING ME
CRAZY NOW AND I THINK IT'S TURNING
THE INSIDE EDGES OF MY TEETH, THE
PART I CAN'T GET AT WITH BRUSHES OR
FLOSS, INTO A CORAL REEF THAT IS WEARING
AWAY THE SIDES OF MY TONGUE. IT'S A
VICIOUS CYCLE. I'M COUNTING ON EVERYTHING
HOLDING TOGETHER IN SOME FASHION FOR
ANOTHER 120 HOURS. AFTER THAT I'LL TAKE MY
CHANCES.

I WOULD SO LOVE NOT TO EAT ANY THING FOR A DAY. NOT BECAUSE (NOT ONLY BECAUSE) EATING IS SO PAINFUL, BUT JUST BECAUSE THE OBLIGATION OF EATING ALL THOSE CALORIES EVERY DAY IS DRIVING ME CRAZY... I DREAM ABOUT CALORIES, AND DIFFERENT COMBINATIONS OF OILS, MILK, ENSURE, BENECALORIES THAT WILL GIVE ME DIFFERENT CALORIE COUNTS. I NOW HAVE MY OWN HR RECORD AS IT WERE: THIS MORNING I HAD A 1880 CALORIE MILK SHAKE. OBVIOUSLY THE 2000 CALORIE SHAKE BECKONS JUST OVER THE HORIZON.

ROBERT "GUZZLER" GOMEZ DRANK 7 ENSURES IN A SINGLE DAY STILL A RECORD

SPENT THE DAY PAYING FOR THE HUBRIS OF THE MORNING DRINK. THAT LAST 175 CALORIES PUT ME IN A TIZZY I DIDN'T GET OUT OF FOR ABOUT 12 HOURS. THINGS BEGAN WELL ENOUGH. JUDE

GAVE ME A COMPLEX OIL MASSAGE THAT FELT GOOD THOUGH LONG RANGE EFFECTIVENESS

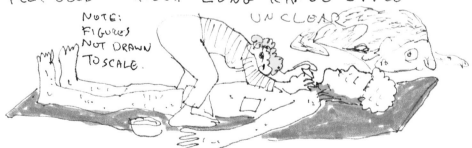

NOTE: FIGURES NOT DRAWN TO SCALE.

UNCLEAR

THEN TOM AND JOSH AND PETER AND FAMILIES CAME OVER AND WE ALL DROVE OUT TO JACK'S PLACE IN BOXFORD TO RETURN THE CAR AND HAVE SOME FUN IN THE COUNTRYSIDE. I THINK WE OVER SOLD THE TRIP TO THE KIDS.

THEY HEARD "FARM" AND WERE
LOOKING FOR LIVESTOCK BEYOND
THE ADORABLE DOGS.
I DON'T THINK THE
GOLDEN BARN WAS
THAT MUCH OF A HIT
IT LOOKED PRETTY
CRAPPY TO TELL
THE TRUTH

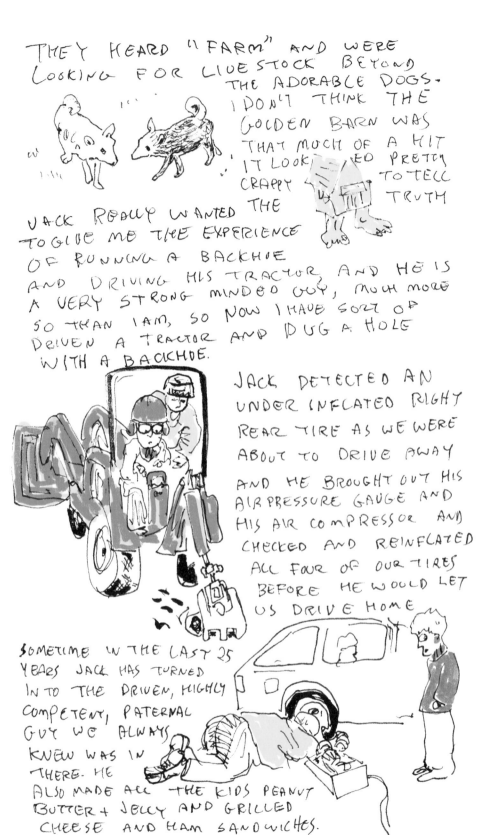

JACK REALLY WANTED
TO GIVE ME THE EXPERIENCE
OF RUNNING A BACKHOE
AND DRIVING HIS TRACTOR, AND HE IS
A VERY STRONG MINDED GUY, MUCH MORE
SO THAN I AM, SO NOW I HAVE SORT OF
DRIVEN A TRACTOR AND DUG A HOLE
WITH A BACKHOE.

JACK DETECTED AN
UNDER INFLATED RIGHT
REAR TIRE AS WE WERE
ABOUT TO DRIVE AWAY
AND HE BROUGHT OUT HIS
AIR PRESSURE GAUGE AND
HIS AIR COMPRESSOR AND
CHECKED AND REINFLATED
ALL FOUR OF OUR TIRES
BEFORE HE WOULD LET
US DRIVE HOME

SOMETIME IN THE LAST 25
YEARS JACK HAS TURNED
INTO THE DRIVEN, HIGHLY
COMPETENT, PATERNAL
GUY WE ALWAYS
KNEW WAS IN
THERE. HE
ALSO MADE ALL THE KIDS PEANUT
BUTTER + JELLY AND GRILLED
CHEESE AND HAM SANDWICHES.

I RAN DOWN THE BATTERY ON MY IPHONE AND WE HAD TO USE THE PRIUS' ANCIENT GPS SYSTEM, WHICH FOR SOME REASON DECIDED TO GUIDE US HOME DOWN THE SMALLEST AND SLOWEST STREETS IN SOMERVILLE AND CAMBRIDGE.

I THINK THIS WAS PERHAPS THE WORST 60 MINUTES OF MY TREATMENT. I PUT MY KNAPSACK WITH ALL MY MEDICATIONS IN THE BACK OF THE CAR AND I SAT THERE BASICALLY MUTE, AS THE STUPID MACHINE KEPT SENDING US DOWN ONE INEFFICIENT STREET AFTER ANOTHER I COULD ONLY SQUEAK LIKE A MOUSE, NOT THAT I WOULD HAVE BEEN MUCH GOOD IF I COULD HAVE SPOKEN. EVERYTHING HURTS, AND NOTHING WORKS. I DRAGGED EVERYONE OUT TO JACK'S HOUSE, THEN I DRAGGED EVERYONE BACK TO MY APARTMENT. THEY'RE ALL DOING EVERYTHING FOR ME BECAUSE THEY LOVE ME AND THEY WANT TO HELP ME GET BETTER, AND I AM TURNING INTO A BUMP ON A LOG. ONLY FOUR MORE DAYS TO GO WITH THIS, AND IN A WAY, THIS IS THE EASY PART. ALL I HAVE TO DO IS ENDURE THE PHYSICAL ORDEAL, AND I'VE DONE MY JOB. IT'S SPECIAL TO BE SICK AT THE HOSPITAL, IT'S NOT SPECIAL TO LIVE WITH BEING SICK WHEN YOU'RE BACK HOME TRYING TO LIVE A NORMAL LIFE. I'M NOT SURE I WILL BE SO GOOD AT THAT.

TONIGHT I REALLY THOUGHT I WAS GOING TO BE UNABLE TO FINISH MY PRIMARY JOB: DRINKING ENSURE SHAKES. I REALLY FELT LIKE THE NEXT BOTTLE I DRANK WOULD COME RIGHT UP LIKE OLD FAITHFUL.

EVERYONE NOW AND I'VE FEEDING TUBE END OF IT'S NOT OF THE NOT THE IT? IT'S

THINKS IT'S OVER WON. I BEAT THE AND THAT'S THE THE STORY. BUT EVEN THE BEGINNING STORY. ACTUALLY, IT'S STORY, AT ALL, IS JUST THE STUPID

CHAPTER OF THE STORY THAT FOCUSES ON THE FEEDING TUBE.

THAT DIDN'T KEEP ME FROM TOR-TURING POOR JUDE AND MOM FOR A COUPLE OF HOURS THIS EVENING AS I PER-FORMED MY BREAK OUT HIT: DRINKING DINNER.

FIRST I SAT IN A DAZE FOR ABOUT AN HOUR MIXED INGREDI-SUPER OFF ANY THIS WAS A JOURNEY ALONE. AFTER I MIXED

I HATE TO SEE MATT NOT BEING MATT

THEN I CAREFULLY ALL THE MAGIC ENTS FOR A SHAKE, WAVING OFFERS TO HELP: I HAD TO TAKE UP THE SHAKE

I SPENT TEN MINUTES PREPARING MY BODY TO DRINK IT: GARGLING, BRUSHING, TAKING SEVERAL PAIN KILLERS AND ANTI-NAUSEA ~~PILLS A~~ PILLS, BRUSHING, FLOSSING. JUDE WENT TO LIE DOWN. I CLEARED A PATH THROUGH THE APARTMENT SO I COULD WALK OFF THE PAIN AS I DRANK. I GOT IT DOWN IN ABOUT TEN SWALLOWS. AND I DIDN'T THROW UP. NOT QUITE MY 4000 AVERAGE BUT PRETTY CLOSE. NOW I'M FEELING PRETTY GOOD ABOUT MYSELF.

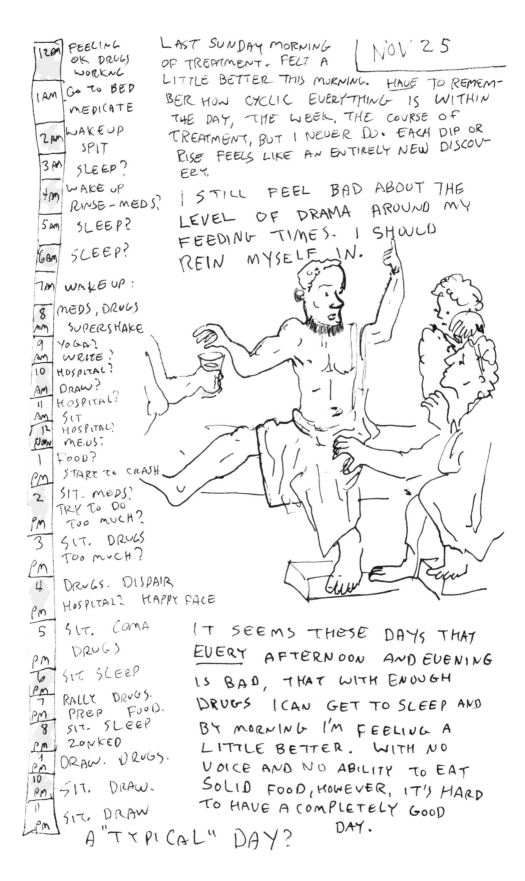

Time column (left):

12AM FEELING OK DRUGS WORKNG
1AM GO TO BED MEDICATE
2AM WAKE UP SPIT
3AM SLEEP?
4AM WAKE UP RINSE - MEDS?
5AM SLEEP?
6AM SLEEP?
7AM WAKE UP:
8 AM MEDS, DRUGS SUPERSHAKE
9 AM YOGA? WRITE?
10 AM HOSPITAL? DRAW?
11 AM HOSPITAL? SIT
12 NOON HOSPITAL! MEDS?
1 PM FOOD? START TO CRASH
2 PM SIT. MEDS? TRY TO DO TOO MUCH?
3 PM SIT. DRUGS TOO MUCH?
4 PM DRUGS. DISPAIR HOSPITAL? HAPPY FACE
5 PM SIT. COMA DRUGS
6 PM SIT. SLEEP
7 PM RALLY DRUGS. PREP FOOD.
8 PM SIT. SLEEP ZONKED
9 PM DRAW. DRUGS.
10 PM SIT. DRAW.
11 PM SIT. DRAW

A "TYPICAL" DAY?

LAST SUNDAY MORNING OF TREATMENT. FELT A LITTLE BETTER THIS MORNING. HAVE TO REMEMBER HOW CYCLIC EVERYTHING IS WITHIN THE DAY, THE WEEK, THE COURSE OF TREATMENT, BUT I NEVER DO. EACH DIP OR RISE FEELS LIKE AN ENTIRELY NEW DISCOVERY.

NOV 25

I STILL FEEL BAD ABOUT THE LEVEL OF DRAMA AROUND MY FEEDING TIMES. I SHOULD REIN MYSELF IN.

IT SEEMS THESE DAYS THAT EVERY AFTERNOON AND EVENING IS BAD, THAT WITH ENOUGH DRUGS I CAN GET TO SLEEP AND BY MORNING I'M FEELING A LITTLE BETTER. WITH NO VOICE AND NO ABILITY TO EAT SOLID FOOD, HOWEVER, IT'S HARD TO HAVE A COMPLETELY GOOD DAY.

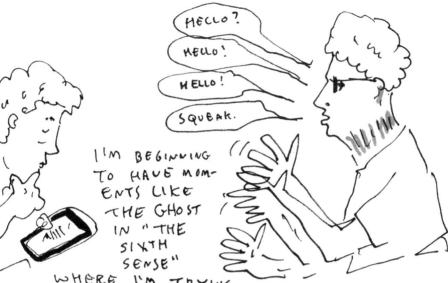

HELLO?

HELLO!

HELLO!

SQUEAK.

I'M BEGINNING TO HAVE MOMENTS LIKE THE GHOST IN "THE SIXTH SENSE" WHERE I'M TRYING TO TALK TO SOMEONE AND THEY CAN'T HEAR ME. I KEEP REPEATING MYSELF BUT I CAN'T GET ANY LOUDER AND IF NO ONE SEES ME FLUTTERING MY HANDS THEN NO ONE KNOWS I'M TRYING TO COMMUNICATE FINALLY I SIMPLY BEGIN TO SQUEAK.

TURNS OUT, THERE REALLY ISN'T THAT MUCH I NEED TO TELL PEOPLE ANYHOW. DOES ANYONE NEED TO KNOW THE LEAD PROTAGONIST IN CATCH-22?

AFTER MY BIG START YESTERDAY, I DROPPED BEHIND THE 4000 CALORIE ARMS RACE FOR THE FIRST TIME IN OVER A WEEK. SINCE THIS IS REALLY ALL I THINK ABOUT NOW, THIS FAILURE HAS COMMENTATORS BUZZING: THE FIRST INDICATIONS OF A SYSTEMS WIDE COLLAPSE OR A HEALTHY AND INEVITABLE MARKET READJUSTMENT? TODAY'S INTAKE CLOCKED IN AT 4040, OVER THE MAGIC STANDARD, BUT NOT ROBUSTLY SO. IT WOULD SEEM THAT FREEDMAN IS PLAYING OUT A CAUTIOUS END GAME STRATEGY, CONSUMING JUST ENOUGH CALORIES TO SILENCE HIS CRITICS

WHO WARN OF A MASSIVE FAILURE AND A RETURN TO SOVIET STYLE GASTRIC TUBE ARTIFICIAL INFLATION OF THE MARKET. I CAN NO LONGER TELL WHAT IS FOOD, PHLEGM OR MEDICINE. EVERYTHING HAS ABOUT THE SAME GOOEY TEXTURE.

THE MAGIC MOUTHWASH I SWIG AND GARGLE 20 HOURS A DAY IS EXACTLY THE SAME AS THE CLEAR GOO AND THE YELLOW WADS I HAWK UP FROM THE BACK OF MY THROAT, ONLY IT'S PINK. THE SUPER SHAKES, ONCE THE SAFFLOWER AND OLIVE OILS AND THE HEAVY CREAM AND THE LITTLE SAUCERS OF BENE CALORIES ARE MIXED IN, IS THE SAME. I CAN'T TELL WHAT'S COMING OR GOING.

THIS EVENING I TRIED TO KISS NINA GOODBYE. BUT A STRAND OF SALIVA, AS STRONG AND RESILIENT AS THE WEB GOO THAT SHOOTS OUT OF SPIDER-MAN'S WRISTS, BLOCKED US. SHE HAD TO DUCK AWAY AND GIVE ME A LITTLE PECK ON THE CHEEK

GOOD NIGHT MATT

GMPH BGHT

THE STRANGEST CHANGE, THOUGH, IS THE SILENCE I DOUBT I'VE SAID MORE THAN TWO DOZEN WORDS ALL DAY. IF I CAN'T TALK, WHO AM I? IF I CAN'T EAT, WHAT AM I?

THE LESS I CAN EAT, THE MORE
EATING FASCINATES ME. WHEN I
WAS A COLLEGE FRESHMAN LOSING WEIGHT
FOR LIGHTWEIGHT CREW, I NOTICED I WAS
IDLY DOODLING PICTURES OF FATTY
FOODS IN MY NOTE BOOKS.

I HAD A THING
FOR CHOCOLATE
ECLAIRS. THEY LIKED SERVING
THEM AT THE DINING HALLS, AND I HATED
TO MISS THEM, EVEN IF I WAS ON A HIGHLY
RESTRICTED DIET. TURNS OUT YOU CAN
LOSE WEIGHT AND STILL EAT CHOCOLATE
ECLAIRS, IF YOU EAT NOTHING ELSE.

TONIGHT WHILE HAMMERING DOWN THE
LAST, PARTICULARLY PAINFUL SHAKE
OF THE DAY, I READ THE DINING SEC-
TION OF THE NY TIMES, WHICH THESE
DAYS IS PARTICULARLY TAKEN WITH MEAT
AND CHEESE AND WINE.

GOAT

ALL THAT
WAS LEFT
FROM A
GOAT WAS
THE LIVER
AND A LEG

"I CHOSE THE LIVER"

LIVER

RUSTIC FRENCH
SAUCE OF VERMOUTH
AND LARDONS

MESS OF CARMELIZED
ONIONS

"STAGGERINGLY
HEARTY"

CUSHION OF MASHED
POTATOES

CHICKEN PASTILLA

DUSTING
OF CON-
FECTIONERS
SUGAR

PHYLLO DOUGH
SHREDDED CHICKEN
QUAIL'S EGGS, SAFFRON
CINNAMON AND HONEY
ALMOND PASTE

WEEK. I WILL BE RELYING ON A LOT OF "LASTS" TO GET ME THROUGH THE NEXT THREE DAYS. I'M ON FUMES NOW. WAS UP THREE OF FOUR TIMES LAST NIGHT WITH MOUTH PAIN. CAN'T GET AWAY FROM IT NOW. MY MOUTH IS PERMANENTLY METAL FLAVORED, DRY AND PAINFULLY SLICED UP DID SOME SUN SALUTATIONS BUT COULDN'T GET FAR. FORCED A FEW CORE EXERCISES, DITTO I'M LIGHT HEADED NOW AND I THINK I REALLY COULD LOSE MY BALANCE IF I DIDN'T WATCH IT HAVING TROUBLE DRAWING THE DIZZY LINES!

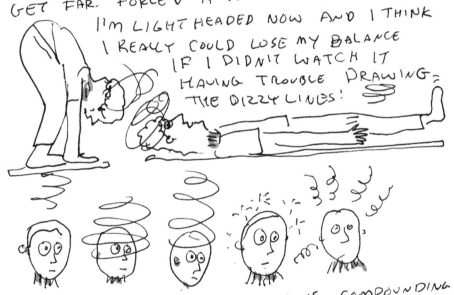

DOING THIS ALL IN SILENCE IS COMPOUNDING THE PROBLEM. WHEN YOU CAN'T TALK ABOUT ANYTHING CASUALLY OR IN THE ABSTRACT, THERE IS NO RELEASE VALUE. EVERYTHING PILES UP. NOUNS AND GESTURES GET BASIC INFORMATION ACROSS, BUT NOT MUCH ELSE. AND IT'S CATCHING MOM AND I TOOK A WALK AND SHE WANTED ME TO SEE HOW ELEGANTLY A TREE WAS GROWING OUT OF THE GROUND. SHE POINTED WITH ONE HAND TO THE TRUNK AND PUMPED WITH HER OTHER FIST. SO MAYBE ABSTRACT QUALITIES CAN BE COMMUNICATED NONVERBALLY.

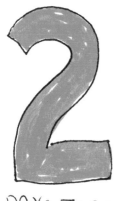

2

DAYS TO GO

I TOLD JOSH I WAS FEELING LIGHTHEADED AND HE SAID, "YOU'RE DEHYDRATED"

WHEN I FEEL LIGHTHEADED, I UNDERSTAND IT AS THE FIRST OVERT MANIFESTATION OF AN ONRUSHING AND UNAVOIDABLE CATASTROPHE, LIKE THE FIRST TIME THE HEROINE COUGHS IN A LOVE STORY AND YOU KNOW SHE'S GOING TO DIE IN THE LAST SCENE IN A HOSPITAL ROOM SURROUNDED BY FLOWERS AND LOVED ONES.

WHEN JOSH HEARS "LIGHTHEADED" HE GOES TO WORK TO FIND A DOCTOR WHO WILL GIVE ME SOME IV AND PUMP ME BACK INTO SHAPE

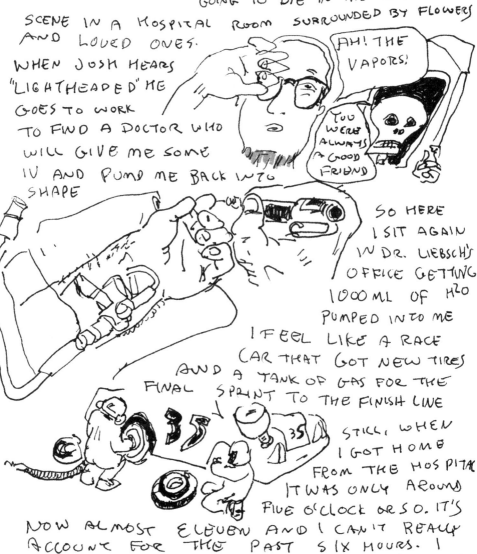

AH! THE VAPORS!

YOU WERE ALWAYS A GOOD FRIEND

SO HERE I SIT AGAIN IN DR. LIEBSCH'S OFFICE GETTING 1000 ML OF H2O PUMPED INTO ME

I FEEL LIKE A RACE CAR THAT GOT NEW TIRES AND A TANK OF GAS FOR THE FINAL SPRINT TO THE FINISH LINE

STILL, WHEN I GOT HOME FROM THE HOSPITAL IT WAS ONLY AROUND FIVE O'CLOCK OR SO. IT'S NOW ALMOST ELEVEN AND I CAN'T REALLY ACCOUNT FOR THE PAST SIX HOURS. I DID DRINK MY CALORIES, BUT OTHER THAN THAT, I THINK I HAVE JUST BEEN SITTING STILL

IT'S CLOSE ENOUGH NOW THAT I HOPE TO DRAG MYSELF OVER THE FINISH LINE USING "THIS IS THE LAST TIME" TYPE MILESTONES AS MOTIVATION AND AS A MEANS OF KEEPING ATTENTION FOCUSED ON SMALL DETAILS, THUS AVOIDING THE DESTABILIZING DISTRACTION OF ABSTRACT, I.E. IMAGINATIVE, REASONING. WHICH

TURNS OUT TO BE JUST AS COUNTER PRODUCTIVE WHEN TRYING TO SURVIVE CANCER THERAPY AS IT IS WHEN ONE IS TRYING TO PERFORM AN ATHLETIC TASK OR CREATE AN INTERESTING WORK OF ART

TWO MORE MORNINGS OF SUPER SHAKES. TWO MORE SESSIONS ON THE TABLE TRYING NOT TO THROW UP. TWO MORE TIMES TO PRY OPEN MY MOUTH AND STUFF THE BITE BLOCK IN.

AT FIRST, IT WAS NO PROBLEM GETTING THE BLOCK IN

DAY 1

ABOUT HALF WAY THROUGH I NOTICED MY MOUTH WASN'T OPENING QUITE SO WELL

DAY 17

WHOP!

NOW I HAVE TO PRAC- TICALLY HAMMER THE THING IN

DAY 33

THE PLASTIC BURNS AND TINGLES ON THE ROOF OF MY MOUTH AND THE TOP OF MY TONGUE. MY LIPS GO INTO SPASM AND SIZZLE WHEN THE RADIATION IS SWITCHED ON. PRETTY ~~PROUD OF~~ NOT FREAKING TO DEATH DURING RADIATION. I'VE GOTTEN GOOD ABOUT OUT ABOUT CHOKING RADIATION. I'M BASICALLY IN A COMA. I'M PRETTY SURE I CAN CLEAR THE DECKS AND SLEEP THROUGH TWO MORE SESSIONS

I'M GETTING MORE OBSESSED WITH FOOD I THINK, EVEN AS I FEEL AS THOUGH I AM FURTHER AND FURTHER AWAY FROM EATING SOLID FOOD AGAIN. I JUST WANT TO CHEW SOMETHING AND SWALLOW IT AND NOT JUST CHOKE DOWN ANOTHER THICK VISCOUS LIQUID (WHY HAVEN'T I BECOME TOTALLY NAUSEATED BY THE MERE SIGHT OF ENSURE? I MUST REALLY LOVE TO EAT).

THE GUYS IN THE SONIC COMMERCIALS SEEM TO BE REALLY ENJOYING THEIR FOOD. I WANT TO SIT IN A CAR AND EAT JUNK FOOD.

DAY 34

SO THIS IS PRETTY NOV 27

SERIOUS NOW. THE SECOND TO LAST DAY. ALMOST DONE. WHICH MAKES EVERY ACHE AND PAIN ALL THE SCARIER. THIS MORNING I HAD MY MOST DIFFICULTY SWALLOW- ING PILLS YET - SUPPOSE

THAT SHUTS DOWN. AND NOW I DETECT A PAIN ON MY LOWER RIGHT SIDE. NEAR A KIDNEY? ARE MY KIDNEYS SHUTTING DOWN? OR IS IT MUSCLE PAIN? WAS IT THAT LITTLE SPAT OF YOGA YESTERDAY? DID I PULL SOME- THING?

BIG MEETINGS TODAY. JOSH IS GOING TO SEE THE FOUNDER OF THE ADENOID CYSTIC CARCINOMA RESEARCH FOUNDATION. MY FAMILY IS AMAZING. THEY DON'T SIT AROUND, THEY DO THINGS. I HAVE A FEELING JOSH AND JEFF WILL BE BUDDIES. THEY SOUND VERY SIMILAR. AFTER MY THERAPY I HAVE AN (ALMOST) EXIT MEETING WITH DR LIEBSCH WHEREIN WE ORGANIZE MY FIRST WEEKS POST TREATMENT FOR WEANING ME OFF MY PAIN MEDICATION AND GETTING BACK ON REAL FOOD. THAT COULD TAKE AWHILE. IT'S GOING TO BE VERY STRANGE, NOT HAVING ANY STRUCTURE AROUND MY DAYS AND NO FORM TO MY

ANTI-CANCER PROGRAM. I'M JUST
GOING TO BE SITTING AT HOME
FOR AWHILE I GUESS. I'LL

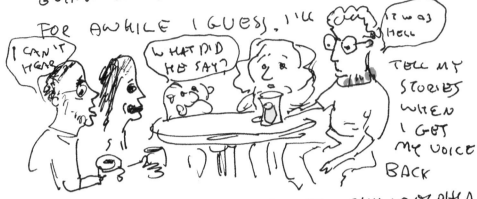

WILL I BE ABLE TO GO TO PHILADELPHIA
TO SEE MY STUDENTS? I HOPE SO. BUT
I'M NOT SURE ABOUT THAT 72 HOUR
ORDEAL THEY HAVE FOR THEIR FINAL
CRITIQUES. MAYBE I CAN SLEEP IN
THE BACK OF THE ROOM

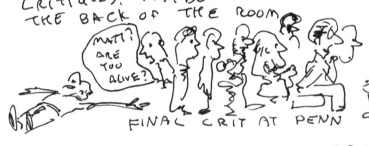

FINAL CRIT AT PENN

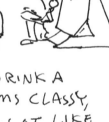

NOW I WANT TO DRINK A
MANHATTAN. SEEMS CLASSY,
ALSO IT LOOKS A LOT LIKE
THE ROXICET I'VE BEEN
SWILLING FOR WEEKS
EXCEPT YOU CAN PUT BOURBON OR
BRANDIED CHERRIES OR VERMOUTH OR
APRICOT LIQUEUR OR BITTERS OR ANY-
THING ELSE YOU WANTED IN IT. OF COURSE
IT TURNS OUT THE RECIPE WRITER WHO
ENTICED ME DRINKS THEM IN HONOR
OF HER DEAD HUSBAND, WHO WAS A
MANHATTAN MAN BEFORE HE PASSED
AWAY DUE TO CANCER IN 2010. DAMN.

THE NEXT-TO-LAST DAY WENT BY IN PRETTY GOOD FASHION. JOSH MET WITH THE GUY WHO FOUNDED ACC RESEARCH AND THEY BEGAN TO PUT TOGETHER THE BEGINNING OF MY SECOND STAGE OF WAR AGAINST THE TUMOR. CHECK. ALL I'M DOING IS WORRYING ABOUT ENERGY SHAKES AND A PROGRAM TO SAVE MY LIFE IS BEING CONSTRUCTED.

READY? AIM...

NEVER HAVE SO FEW OWED SO MUCH TO SO MANY. BY THE TIME **ALL** THE TIME AND ENERGY AND GOOD WILL AND NATURAL AND HUMAN RESOURCES THAT HAVE BEEN EXPENDED ON MY BEHALF HAVE BEEN ADDED, THE PUNDITS MUST ASK, HAS IT BEEN WORTH IT? IS THIS MAN WORTH THE EFFORT!

YES!

NO!

I GUESS IT'S A CABLE TV DEBATE TOPIC.

LUCKILY NO ONE ASKS ME MY OPINION AND I CAN GO ABOUT MY BUSINESS BEING SO GRATEFUL TO EVERYONE AROUND ME BUT UNABLE TO PUT MY FEELINGS INTO WORDS. INSTEAD I MADE THOSE STUPID LITTLE FIGURES FOR SOME OF THE PEOPLE WHO HELPED ME. I DON'T THINK THEY WENT OVER ALL THAT WELL

I'LL TRY NOT TO TAKE THIS PERSONALLY

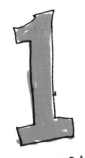

1

MORE DAY
TO GO.

So EVERYTHING I DO TONIGHT I DO FOR THE LAST TIME AS A CANCER PATIENT UNDERGOING CHEMO AND RADIATION TREATMENT. MY STORY IS JUST ABOUT DONE AND MY 'EXPERIENCE' SUCH AS IT IS ALREADY EXPERIENCED. I SUPPOSE THE "REAL" STORY, THE ONE I WILL BEGIN HONING AND PERFECTING ON THURSDAY, THE DAY <u>AFTER</u> TREATMENT ENDS STILL IS YET TO BE WRITTEN, BUT THAT'S WHY I'M PLEASED TO HAVE ALMOST COMPLETED THIS LITTLE BOOK. IT DEFINITELY BECAME PART OF THE STORY- I THOUGHT ABOUT WHAT WOULD GO IN IT AND NOT GO IN IT, AND IT GAVE ME AS PRACTICAL AND AS REAL A DISTRACTION FROM THE CHALLENGES OF THE TREATMENT AS MY CALORIE COUNTING AND SYMPTOM MONITORING HABITS EVER DID, BUT I HOPE IT WILL KEEP THE "REAL" STORY HONEST. I'M A LITTLE AFRAID IT WILL BE ALL BUT INCOHERENT AND EVEN TOO GRUMPY FOR ANYONE BUT ME TO EVER READ, BUT IT IS A DAY BY DAY ACCOUNTING OF MY BLIND STUMBLING FOR- WARD INTO THE UNKNOWN OF THIS TREAT- MENT. DR. LIEBSCH ASKED IF THERE WAS ANYTHING FROM MY EXPERIENCE WITH THIS TREATMENT PROGRAM THAT I THOUGHT WOULD HELP SOMEBODY ELSE IN THE SAME POSITION AND I REALIZED I REALLY WASN'T SURE THERE WAS-(I ALSO REALIZED I COULDN'T PUT IT INTO WORDS WITH A BROKEN MOUTH) EVERYONE'S EXPERIENCE IS UNIQUE AND ALSO JUST LIKE EVERYONE ELSE'S. WE BOTH OWN AND SHARE THIS HISTORY WITH EVERYBODY.

DAY 35

HERE IT IS FINALLY. THE

LAST DAY OF TREATMENT. JOSH AND FAMILY HAVE ALREADY TAKEN OFF FOR L.A. MOM HAS ALREADY DONE ALL HER MORNING EXERCISES.

I'VE ALEADY HAD MY FIRST 1825 CALORIES OF THE DAY. I'LL NEED A RECORD DAY OF DRINKING TO GET MY AVERAGE BACK UP TO THE MAGIC 4000 AVE.

EVERYTHING IS IN PLACE FOR A PRETTY SMOOTH DAY EXCEPT FOR MY TONGUE, WHICH IS ACTING UP.

THE LAST SESSION PASSED WITHOUT INCIDENT

THE TREATMENT STAFF GAVE ME A CERTIFICATE AND A PIN

MATT PROBOOM
3MM 6MM
10MM GRAY

I RANG THE BELL

RING THIS BELL THREE TIMES WELL ITS TOLL WILL CLEARLY SAY MY TREATMENTS ARE DONE THIS COURSE HAS RUN AND NOW I'M ON MY WAY.

I THINK MOM LIKED THIS MORE THAN MY HIGH SCHOOL GRADUATION

DO YOU HAVE A CLEAN SHIRT FOR THE VIDEO?

HAWB!

JUDY BROUGHT EVERYONE A HUGE BOX OF PASTRIES

I HANDED OUT THE LAST OF MY LITTLE GOLD PEOPLE. ONE CASUALTY ALREADY, NOTHING SUPER GLUE CAN'T FIX

LITTLE IV MAN FELL CRACK!

WHILE BIG IV MAN WAS GETTING IV.

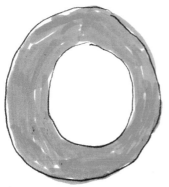

DAYS LEFT
TO GO. THAT'S
IT. I'M DONE

THEY DID END UP CANCELLING THE FINAL CHEMOTHERAPY SESSION AFTER ALL. THEY ONLY KEEP IT AS AN OPTION IF THERE ARE TWO OR MORE RADIATION SESSIONS LEFT AFTER THE LAST AND THEY WERE HEDGING THEIR BETS SO I'M JUST GETTING WATER TO PLUMP ME UP.

I'M SORT OF IN A PICKLE HERE. ON ENOUGH MEDS THAT I DROP IN AND OUT OF THE WORLD FOR 30-60 MINUTES AT A TIME, BUT NOTHING STOPS THIS TONGUE FROM HURTING.

NOTHING CAN OPEN UP THE LITTLE I HAVE TO GET NUTRIENTS

AND OPEN TINY PASSAGE ALL THE THROUGH

I ASKED KATE THE NURSE IF ANY-ONE GETS THROUGH THIS KIND OF RADIATION WITHOUT NARCOTICS. AT FIRST SHE SAYS "NO", BUT THEN SHE SAYS, ONCE A YEAR OR SO SOMEONE GOES THROUGH WITHOUT DRUGS. THERE WAS A

THE MEDICAL PEOPLE SAY "DRUG UP" - SPEND THE REST OF THIS ORDEAL AS OUT OF IT AS POSSIBLE. BUT I SORT OF WANT TO BE AWARE OF WHAT'S HAPPENING. BESIDES I DON'T THINK ANYTHING WILL REALLY BLUNT THE TONGUE.

THAT'S OKAY HONEY. GOD TAKES REALLY GOOD CARE OF ME

LITTLE OLD LADY "80 POUNDS" NOTHING WHOSE FACE WAS MELTING OFF FROM THE RADIATION. BUT SHE SAID THE SAME THING EVERY TIME THEY OFFERED HER SOME DRUGS. "SHE HYPNOTIZED HERSELF" SAID MY MOTHER

SHE'S LIKE MY NEIGHBOR PERLENE, THE CHURCH LADY. IN PERL'S WORLD THERE IS NO SUCH THING AS LUCK. IT'S ALL GOD'S WILL.

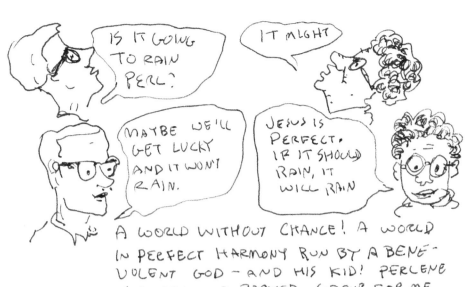

IS IT GOING TO RAIN PERL?

IT MIGHT

MAYBE WE'LL GET LUCKY AND IT WON'T RAIN.

JESUS IS PERFECT. IF IT SHOULD RAIN, IT WILL RAIN

A WORLD WITHOUT CHANCE! A WORLD IN PERFECT HARMONY RUN BY A BENE-VOLENT GOD—AND HIS KID! PERLENE IS LEADING A PRAYER GROUP FOR ME. SO I GOT THAT GOING ON.

ON THE RADIO I HEARD A LETTER VAN GOGH WROTE TO THE WIFE OF THE CAFE OWNER IN ARLES WHEN HE HEARD SHE WAS SICK.

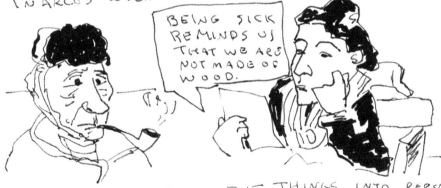

BEING SICK REMINDS US THAT WE ARE NOT MADE OF WOOD.

A LONG TIME AGO, AT THE BEGINING OF MY TREATMENT, JUDE ASKED ME IF I THOUGHT BEING SICK MADE ME MORE AWARE OF THE WONDER-FULLNESS OF LIFE. I DIDN'T SAY YES BECAUSE I HAD NEVER THOUGHT IN THOSE TERMS TO BEGIN WITH, AND NOW I THINK I WAS TOO SCARED OF DYING TO START TO

PUT THINGS INTO PERSPEC-TIVE—AS IF THAT WOULD BE A STEP TOWARDS ACCEPT-ING MY SITUATION. I'M MORE OF A WOOD GUY THAN A GOD GUY. BUT I CAN'T DENY ALL THE HELP I'VE RECEIVED HAS CHANGED THE WAY I THINK IN A VERY PRO-FOUND WAY

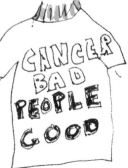

CANCER BAD PEOPLE GOOD

I GOT THE BIG COUNTDOWN TODAY FOR THE END OF TREATMENT, BUT I'M SO USED TO KEEPING MY EYES ON THE GROUND I CAN'T CHANGE THE HABIT: NOW I'M WORRIED ABOUT THE NEXT TWO WEEKS WHEN MY SYMPTOMS STAY BAD BUT THE DRAMA OF THERAPY IS OVER. ALL THE SUPPORT STARTS TO DRY UP. TALK ABOUT FINDING THE GLASS HALF EMPTY! ONE GOOD SIGN ALREADY THOUGH THEY'VE STOPPED ZAPPING MY NECK DIRECTLY FOR A WEEK OR SO, AND THE MAP OF RUSSIA IS GONE. IT'S KIND OF SOFT AND HAIRLESS, LIKE A BABY'S BOTTOM, MY NECK

175 CALORIES

IT'S A LITTE DARK

A LITTLE RED

= (}) = OK

SO MAYBE I'M A QUICK HEALER, THE WOLVERINE OF CANCER PATIENTS

AS FOR THE EXCITING RACE TO SEE IF I COULD FINISH MY TREATMENT AVERAGING OVER THE MAGIC 4000 CALORIE LEVEL, I BEGAN THE DAY AVERAGING 3,988.5 CALORIES, WHICH ROUNDS TO 3,989, GOOD, GREAT, EVEN, BUT NOT A NUMBER TO CONJURE BY. TO REACH 4000 FOR THE TREATMENT SEASON, I WOULD HAVE TO DRINK CLOSE TO MY ALL-TIME DAILY RECORD OF 4270 CALORIES. I WOULD HAVE TO DOWN 4230! COULD I DO IT? I TOP OFF THAT STRONG MORNING PERFORMANCE BY FORCING DOWN 1400 CALORIES AT LUNCH AND DURING 2 HOURS ON IV. THEN PULLED IT HOME WITH A 1045 DINNER FOR A RECORD TYING 4270 DAY AND A SEASON AVERAGE OF 4001.9, WHICH ROUNDS TO 4002!

DRINK UP KIDS

I'M A WINNER AT LAST

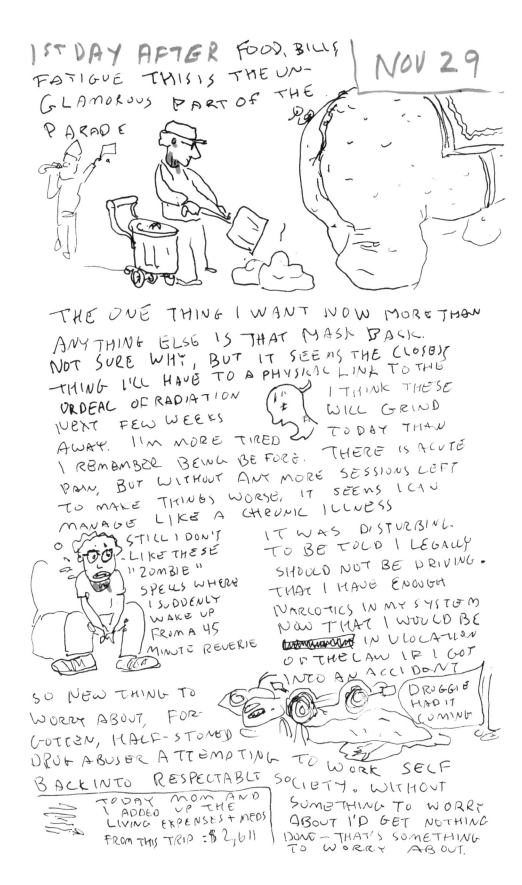

1ST DAY AFTER FOOD, BILLS, FATIGUE THIS IS THE UN-GLAMOROUS PART OF THE PARADE

NOV 29

THE ONE THING I WANT NOW MORE THAN ANYTHING ELSE IS THAT MASK BACK. NOT SURE WHY, BUT IT SEEMS THE CLOSEST THING I'LL HAVE TO A PHYSICAL LINK TO THE ORDEAL OF RADIATION NEXT FEW WEEKS AWAY. I'M MORE TIRED I THINK THESE WILL GRIND TODAY THAN I REMEMBER BEING BEFORE. THERE IS ACUTE PAIN, BUT WITHOUT ANY MORE SESSIONS LEFT TO MAKE THINGS WORSE, IT SEEMS I CAN MANAGE LIKE A CHRONIC ILLNESS

STILL I DON'T LIKE THESE "ZOMBIE" SPELLS WHERE I SUDDENLY WAKE UP FROM A 45 MINUTE REVERIE

IT WAS DISTURBING TO BE TOLD I LEGALLY SHOULD NOT BE DRIVING. THAT I HAVE ENOUGH NARCOTICS IN MY SYSTEM NOW THAT I WOULD BE ~~IN VIOLATION~~ IN VIOLATION OF THE LAW IF I GOT INTO AN ACCIDENT

SO NEW THING TO WORRY ABOUT, FOR-GOTTEN, HALF-STONED DRUG ABUSER ATTEMPTING TO WORK SELF BACK INTO RESPECTABLE SOCIETY. WITHOUT SOMETHING TO WORRY ABOUT I'D GET NOTHING DONE — THAT'S SOMETHING TO WORRY ABOUT.

DRUGGIE HAD IT COMING

TODAY MOM AND I ADDED UP THE LIVING EXPENSES + MEDS FROM THIS TRIP = $2,611

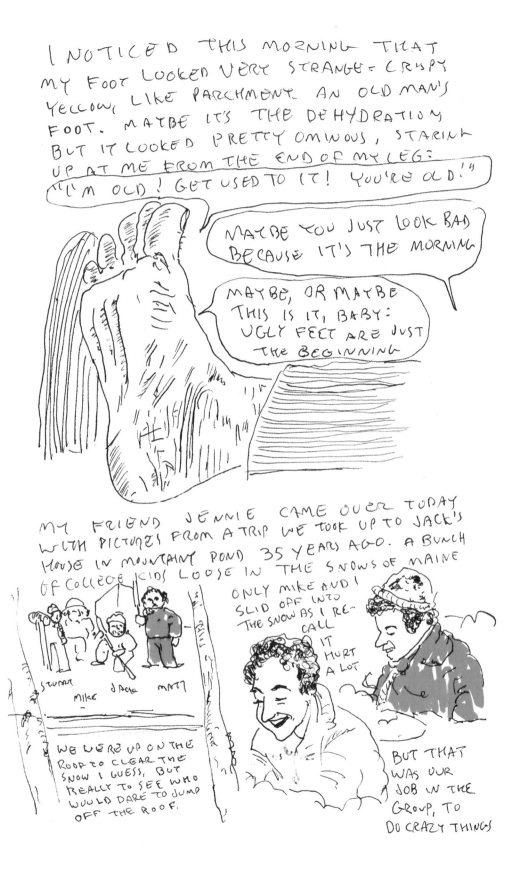

SHE ALSO REVEALED A STRANGE LINK BETWEEN OUR FAMILIES: HER GREAT GRAND FATHER WAS THE MAN BEHIND THE ICONIC NEW ENGLAND SOFT DRINK MOXIE, MY FATHERS FAVORITE DRINK.

DRINK MOXIE

THAT MY FATHER, A VERY SERIOUS MAN, EVEN LIKED A SOFT DRINK, WAS A HUGE DISCOVERY. WHENEVER HE FOUND A BOTTLE, IT WAS TREATED LIKE GOLD. SOMETIMES ONLY HE GOT TO DRINK IT. SOMETIMES WE GOT PRECIOUS LITTLE SIPS. IT DIDN'T MATTER WHAT IT TASTED LIKE, IT WAS AN ELIXIR OF THE GODS. HE TOLD ALL THE MOXIE STORIES HE KNOW - FROM "YOU'VE GOT MOXIE" ENTERING THE ENGLISH LANGUAGE TO THE FACT THAT THE GREAT TED WILLIAMS ENDORSED IT

MAKE MINE MOXIE
TED WILLIAMS SAYS
MOXIE

MOXIE — DRINK MOX — MOXIE

THERE WERE EVEN STRANGE MOXIE HORSEMOBILES. THE DRIVER RODE THE HORSE AND STEERED WITH THE WHEEL IN ITS NECK.

THE HORSEMOBILE REMINDS ME OF BRONSON ALCOTT, THE TRASCENDENTALIST WHO FOUNDED THE UTOPIAN COMMUNITY "FRUITLANDS" JUST A FEW MILES AWAY FROM THE NORTH BRIDGE AND THE "SHOT HEARD ROUND THE WORLD!" THE FRUITLANDERS WERE SO AGAINST ENSLAVING ANIMALS THAT NOT ONLY DID THEY NOT USE THEM AS FARM ANIMALS OR EAT THEIR MEAT, BUT THEY WOULDN'T STEAL THEIR MILK OR THEIR WOOL FOR CLOTHES, OR THEIR MANURE FOR FERTILIZER. THEY ALMOST STARVED AND FROZE TO DEATH IN THEIR ONLY YEAR OF EXISTENCE, 1843. WHATEVER EXTREME FOOD RULES THE 1960'S BROUGHT, THE FRUITLANDERS HAD TOPPED OVER 100 YEARS BEFORE

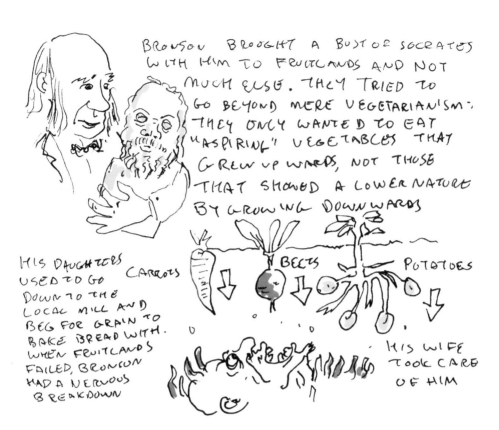

BRONSON BROUGHT A BUST OF SOCRATES WITH HIM TO FRUITLANDS AND NOT MUCH ELSE. THEY TRIED TO GO BEYOND MERE VEGETARIANISM: THEY ONLY WANTED TO EAT "ASPIRING" VEGETABLES THAT GREW UPWARDS, NOT THOSE THAT SHOWED A LOWER NATURE BY GROWING DOWNWARDS

HIS DAUGHTERS USED TO GO DOWN TO THE LOCAL MILL AND BEG FOR GRAIN TO BAKE BREAD WITH. WHEN FRUITLANDS FAILED, BRONSON HAD A NERVOUS BREAKDOWN

CARROTS

BEETS

POTATOES

HIS WIFE TOOK CARE OF HIM

IT'S LATE THURSDAY NIGHT. MY MOTHER HAS GONE TO BED. IN THE MORNING, JUDY WILL TAKE ME TO THE HOSPITAL SO I CAN RECLAIM MY BELOVED MASK AND PICK UP MORE NARCOTICS. THEN JUDE AND OUR FRIEND JOY WILL DRIVE UP HERE FROM NYC. THEN MOM WILL FLY HOME TO CHICAGO. THEN JUDE, JOY, FLEURY AND I WILL DRIVE BACK TO NYC

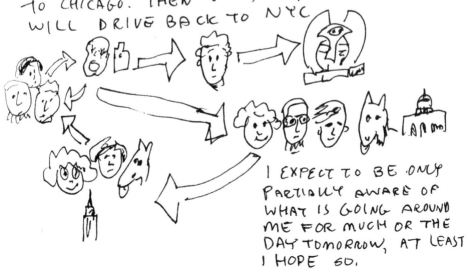

I EXPECT TO BE ONLY PARTIALLY AWARE OF WHAT IS GOING AROUND ME FOR MUCH OR THE DAY TOMORROW, AT LEAST I HOPE SO.

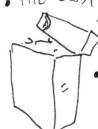

2ND DAY AFTER VARIOUS OMENS | NOV 30

- THE LAST MORNING OF RADIATION THE LAST OF THE WAXED MINT FLAVORED DENTAL TAPE RAN OUT.

- THE DAY AFTER TREATMENT ENDED, I BROKE MY GRADUATION BUTTON: FELL OFF

- LAST NIGHT, I ALMOST SLEPT THROUGH THE NIGHT FOR THE FIRST TIME IN WEEKS JUST A FEW AWAKENINGS FOR SPITTING. NO MEDS. I GUESS I'M HOPING STILL FOR WOLVERINE QUALITY RECOVERY TIMES.

- ON THE OTHER HAND, MY VOICE IS WORSE TODAY THAN EVER. IT'S A SQUEAK.

SQUEAK

WE WENT TO THE HOSPITAL AND RETRIEVED THE MOUTH GUARD AND HELMET. THEY EVEN THREW IN THE NECK SUPPORT TOO. I PUT THE MOUTH GUARD IN JUST TO SEE IF I COULD DO IT — ONLY TWO DAYS DONE A. D I'M ALREADY NOSTALGIC! I'LL NEVER TRY THAT AGAIN — WELL NOT FOR A LONG, LONG TIME. MY JAW FELT LIKE IT WAS ABOUT TO SNAP OFF OF MY SKULL. EVERY PLACE THE GUARD TOUCHED MY TONGUE OR THE ROOF OF MY MOUTH WAS LIKE A RAZOR BLADE STAB. ON SECOND THOUGHT MAYBE I'LL PUT IT IN MY MOUTH EVERY DAY UNTIL IT STOPS HURTING. MY HANDWRITING HAS DETERIORATED BECAUSE I AM IN A CAR NOW DRIVING BACK TO NYC FROM BOSTON.

MOM AND JUDE PULLED OFF THE MATT
TRANSFER WITH NAVY SEAL LIKE PRECISION.
JUDE AND JOY AND FLEUREY ARRIVED
AT ONE. MOM HAD JUST CALLED THE CAB
FOR THE AIRPORT. MOM LEFT AT ONE FIFTEEN.
JOY USED HER SUPER HUMAN PACKING SKILLS
TO FILL THE CAR AND WE WERE GONE BY
TWO.

THE SCENE IN THE CAR,
SOMEWHERE IN WESTERN MASS-
ACHUSETTS

ITS ALMOST 4PM AND GRAY AND SPITTING
SNOW. I THINK WE'RE SOMEWHERE JUST
OUTSIDE HARTFORD. I FEEL LIKE I'M
BEING HAULED BACK TO MY OLD LIFE.
I'VE ALREADY GOTTEN ABOUT TEN
TEXTS FROM MIKE TRYING TO SET UP
MEETINGS NEXT WEEK FOR OUR SHOW.
IN BOSTON I AM SICK AND EVERYONE
TAKES CARE OF ME. IN NEW YORK I
AM CURED AND GETTING ON WITH MY

LIFE. I'M NOT SURE IF EITHER SIT-
UATION IS EXACTLY ACCURATE - MAYBE
I COULD DO A BIT MORE FOR MYSELF,
AND I'M CERTAINLY NOT 100%
AND WON'T BE FOR A LONG TIME.
IT'S GOING TO BE HARD TO
COMMUNICATE THAT TO MY FRIENDS
AND COLLEAGUES THOUGH - THE SAME
ACTING - OUT - MACHISMO THAT HELPED
GET ME THROUGH TEN YEARS OF PAIN
IN MY EAR WITHOUT LOOKING FOR A
REAL DIAGNOSIS IS LIKELY TO HAVE
ME RUNNING AROUND TO MEETINGS AND
OPENINGS AND CLASSES AND MAKING STUFF
IN MY STUDIO LIKE NOTHING BIG
EVER HAPPENED. I WONDER, IF I'M
GOING TO PUT MYSELF IN DANGER.
I GUESS THE MYTHIC FALLING OFF
OF THE CLIFF NEVER QUITE HAPPENED,
THOUGH THERE WERE SEVERAL DAYS
WHEN I THOUGHT IT WAS A<u>BOUT</u> T.
HAPPEN. WHAT NEVER HAPPENED WAS
AN ABSOLUTE AND IRRECONCILABLE & DIS-
CONNECT FROM THE WORLD I WAS FAMILIAR
WITH THAT THREW ME INTO SOME
NEW UNCONTEMPLATED REGION
OF HORROR. DERING,
SO I'M WON CAN SORT
MAYBE I AS LONG
OF GO BACK TO NORMAL. AS LONG
AS I CAN EAT AND SLEEP HOW MUCH
SICKER CAN I GET?
THE VOICE SITUATION IS BAD. THAT
HAS TO GET FIXED BEFORE THINGS
GET BACK TO NORMAL. AND THE
PAIN MEDS. I GUESS I CAN'T GO ON IN A

HAZE LIKE THIS FOREVER. IF I CAN'T DRIVE
I GUESS I CAN'T BE EXPECTED TO MAKE
SENSE IN OTHER, LESS DIRE CIRCUMSTANCES.

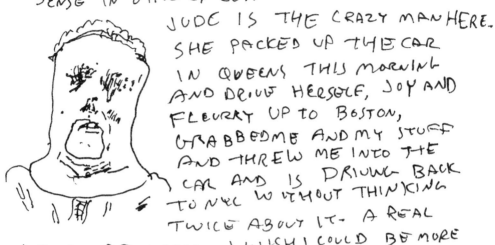

JUDE IS THE CRAZY MAN HERE.
SHE PACKED UP THE CAR
IN QUEENS THIS MORNING
AND DROVE HERSELF, JOY AND
FLEURRY UP TO BOSTON,
GRABBED ME AND MY STUFF
AND THREW ME INTO THE
CAR AND IS DRIVING BACK
TO NYC WITHOUT THINKING
TWICE ABOUT IT. A REAL
WOMAN OF ACTION. I WISH I COULD BE MORE
LIKE HER. IT'S A QUARTER TO FIVE AND ALMOST
DARK IN THE CAR.

RIDGEWOOD. HOME. THEY WENT TO BED.
I TRANSFERED ALL THE PILLS AND MEDICINES
TO THEIR NEW SHELF IN THE KITCHEN.

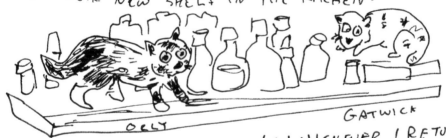

ORLY   GATWICK

I FORGET HOW CHAOTIC NY LOOKS WHENEVER I RETURN,
COMING BACK TRYING TO GET OVER RADIATION IS
GOING TO BE TWICE AS COMPLICATED.
AND WITHOUT A VOICE. JOY INSTINCTIVELY
ANSWERS MY WHISPERS IN A WHISPER OF HER
OWN.   MAYBE TOMORROW I'LL
                              TAKE A WALK, SEE
HELLO   SOME SHOWS, START
HELLO   UNPACKING, GET BACK
OOPS   TO WORK ON SOMETHING.
SORRY
HELLO

3RD DAY AFTER IT'S BEEN A | DEC 1

DAZE. MAYBE THIS IS THE CLIFF
FINALLY. NO MORE ENSURE! EVERYTHING IS A BLOB
IN MY MOUTH. I CAN'T SPEAK. I CAN'T BE UNDER-
STOOD. I SLEPT ALL DAY.

AS IF IN A DREAM I SAW
JUDE AND JOY HAULING OUT
PAPERS AND ORGANIZING BILLS.
THEY DROVE OFF TO HOME
DEPOT AND RETURNED WITH
ENORMOUS BOXES. GARBAGE
CANS FOR
ME TO
SPIT INTO
AND A BRAND
NEW TOILET

THAT WON'T LEAK ALL OVER THE FLOOR EVERY-
TIME IT'S USED.
MY BIG ACCOMPLISHMENT WAS TO DRINK THREE
CUPS OF MISO SOUP. OTHER THAN THAT, NOT MUCH.
I WAS AT LEAST AS MUCH OF A ZOMBIE TODAY
AS I EVER WAS AND I'M A SILENT ONE.
I CAN'T TALK UNLESS I SPEND FIVE
MY MOUTH OF
MINUTES CLEARING I FEND OFF TEXTS FOR
THICK ROPES OF SPIT. I FEND OFF TEXTS FOR
MEETINGS. I WONDER HOW I WILL GET BACK
INTO THE FLOW OF THINGS.
WHEN I STARTED THIS BOOK ON OCTOBER 3
I GAVE MYSELF THE JOB OF FILLING FOUR
PAGES A DAY. ☐☐☐☐ I HAD NO SENSE
THAT I WOULD ACTUALLY GET ANYWHERE, MERELY
THAT THE ASSIGNMENT WOULD LEAVE ME
WITH 240 PAGES OF TEXT AND DRAWINGS
TO SHOW FOR MY TIME GETTING THERAPY,
AND I GUESS I'M GETTING JUST ABOUT WHAT
I BARGAINED FOR: I KEPT TRACK OF WHAT
WAS GOING ON IN MY BODY AND HEAD.

AS BEST I COULD OVER THAT TIME, BUT
NOW IT'S OVER. I THINK I'VE MOVED
FROM ONE ISLAND TO ANOTHER
I DON'T BELIEVE I ACHIEVED
ANY

PRE PROTON   POST PROTON

PARTICULAR WISDOM OR INSIGHT ALONG
THE WAY — NOT THAT I EXPECTED TO — BUT
I GUESS I DID PROVE AT LEAST TO MY OWN
SATISFACTION THAT A CHILDISH TALENT FOR
REMEMBERING AND CELEBRATING THE STATIS-
TICAL MEASURES OF REAL ACHIEVEMENTS
IS IN ITSELF A FORM OF CONCENTRATION
THAT LEADS TO DEDICATED EFFORT

.406   35   4002   .320 12   3.33·1·33†

ALL THOSE NUMBERS AND SEVERAL OTHERS
WILL SERVE NOT JUST AS THE DEVICES TO RE-
MEMBER WHAT I WENT THROUGH, BUT AS
THE SOURCE OF SOME OF THE MORE EMOTIONAL
MEMORIES THEMSELVES.

AND ALL THE PEOPLE WHO HELPED. I WOULDN'T
I COULDN'T SAY HOW MUCH I LOVE AND AM INDEBTED
TO ALL THE PEOPLE WHO HAVE SENT ME NOTES
FED ME, DRIVEN ME, SAT WITH ME, PUT UP WITH
ME IF I HADN'T SPENT THE PREVIOUS PAGES
TRYING TO CONVINCINGLY DEMONSTRATE HOW
UNWORTHY I AM OF ALL THE GOOD THINGS
THAT HAVE COME MY WAY AS A RESULT
OF MY DEVELOPING CANCER. THAT WAS LUCK,
A BOLT OF LIGHTNING AND I CAN'T EVEN
THINK ABOUT IT — A CHANCE EVENT BE-
YOUND THE CALCULATIONS OF PROBA-
BILITY. BUT THE RESPONSE OF MY COMM-
UNITY OF FRIENDS HAD NOTHING TO DO WITH
CHANCE, AND FOR THAT I AM ETERNALLY GRATEFUL.

WELL, WHAT THE FUCK.
I THOUGHT I WAS DONE, DOWN TO THE LAST
PAGE WITH A NICE SEND OFF AND LOOK!
AN EXTRA PAGE. I ACTUALLY ALWAYS
THOUGHT I HAD AN EXTRA TWO PAGES
BUT THEY SEEM(ED) TO HAVE DISAPPEARED
UNTIL I THOUGHT I WAS DONE, THEN
POPPED UP AGAIN AS IF TO SAY,

SERVES ME RIGHT TO
EVEN CONTEMPLATE
A SEARCH FOR MEAN-
ING WHEN I ASSERT
TIME AND TIME AGAIN
THERE IS NO MEANING
ONLY PEOPLE AND
ANIMALS HELPING EACH
OTHER THROUGH THE
CHAOS

RANDOM
CHANCES
WITH THE
UNIVERSE?
I'LL GIVE
YOU TWO
MORE TO
PAGES TO
FILL. HOW'S
THAT FOR RANDOM?

SO IT'S LATE

GATWICK IS SLEEPING ON
MY FATHER'S OLD
PSYCHOANALYTIC COUCH.
ONLY SHE JUST OPENED
HER EYES TO → LOOK
AT ME!

JOY SLEEPS AMIDST ALL THE
BOXES OF STUFF SHE BOUGHT AT HOME DEPOT.

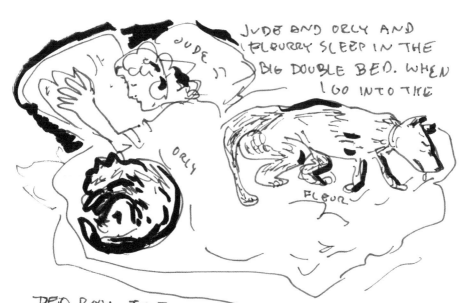

JUDE AND ORLY AND
FLEURRY SLEEP IN THE
BIG DOUBLE BED. WHEN
I GO INTO THE

JUDE

ORLY

FLEUR

BED ROOM TO TRY TO DRAW THEM IN THE
DARKNESS, THEY ALL STIR AND LOOK AT
ME FOR A MOMENT, THEN FALL BACK TO
SLEEP. I HAVE TO TAKE A SHOWER, PUT ON
A FRESH TRANSDERMAL PAIN PATCH AND
TAKE MY NIGHTTIME MEDICATIONS. WHEN
I FINALLY TRY TO CRAWL INTO BED WITH ALL
OF THEM, WITH MY BOX OF TISSUES, MY SPIT-
TOON, MY BOTTLES OF MAGIC MOUTHWASH AND
WATER, IT'S GOING TO BE QUITE A FIGHT.
FLEURRY WILL BARK, ORLY WILL RUN AWAY
AND JUDE WILL TURN OVER. I'LL SNUGGLE
IN AND HOLD HER HAND FOR A BEAUTIFUL
MINUTE OR TWO. THEN I WILL HAVE TO SPIT.

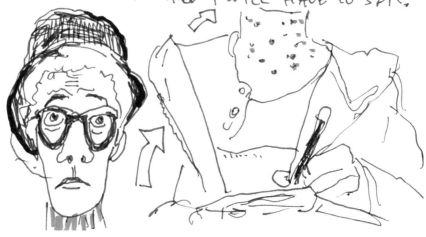

THANKS JUDE DOROTHY BART JOSH JOHANNA
TOM LUKE SAM BEN ELI ABE TEA NOAH MATTY
ABBY SABRINA GABRIEL PAUL MARTINE JUDY HUGH
ALEX ELLEN BILL KATE ANN SARAH BILL BILL
LAURIE BILL PAUL JOHN DENISE BRIAN ERIC DAVID
PAUL DAVID JATIN NANCY NORBERT JIM CAROLINE
KATE DAVID EUNGHO DONNA JON SOONI RICHARD KIM
MIKE JACK MICHICO LARRY ANALIE FRED LARA TOM NOAH
FRANCESCA MONICA JOY JIM VICTORIA ALEX ANN TONI
TERRY JACKIE ORKAN NANY MATT CATHY JANE JONATHAN
VIEVIE MARY BARRIE ALLISON BOB LISA KATHERINE LUISA MARGO
DONNA KAREN LORIE PETER ELI ABE EDEN NATHAN OLLIE CHRISIE
KARBN CRAIG JONATHAN LAURENCE JENNIE PHILLIP DAN
SINA NINA ELIZABETH MEGAN PAVAN TOD ARNIE CHUCK
CHRISEA JULIA FLEURY GATWICK ORLY ALEX FIDO JAMES
JACKIE TESSA SCOTT DAN MANO CAT LAGUARDIA NEWARK
CRYPTON PLUTO SPARKY RENDAN WILL JIM CYNTHIA CATHY
AMBER STEWART DAN LISA DAVID LESLEY GLORIA CAROL
RICHARD BRITTANY SUSAN CHARLES JONATHAN ROBERTA
KATE DAVE ADAM MICHELE JAKE MEGAN MICHAEL
BRENT PAUL RUTH PERLENE FRANK HELEN EDNA TARYN
JONATHAN JANE MARISSA NANCY MICHELLE THOMAS
ARI WARD JOSHUA SARAH MIKE JULIAN MARGOZET
ANNE RACHEL OLIVER DAVID LINDA FRANCES NIKKO
PAUL DAISY CALEB WENDY TODD SUE AVA SUSAN PAULA
CHRIS JANE CHARLOTTE HENTRY LARRY MARY JEFF JOHN MOLLY
JOHN